a wellnes

women of the '60s turning 50

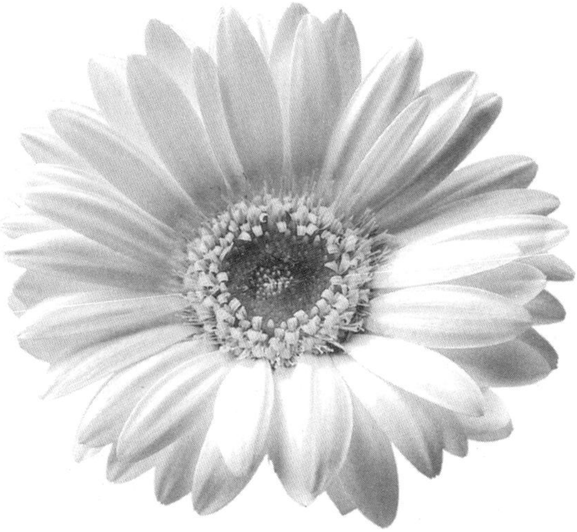

m. sara rosenthal

Prentice Hall Canada
A Pearson Company
Toronto

Canadian Cataloguing in Publication Data

Rosenthal, M. Sara
Women of the '60s turning 50: a wellness guide

Includes index.
ISBN 0-13-026814-3

1. Middle aged women – Health and hygiene. I. Title.

RA778.R673 2000 613'.04244 C00-930132-1

ISBN 0-13-026814-3

Editorial Director, Trade Division: Andrea Crozier
Acquisitions Editor: Nicole de Montbrun
Copy Editor: Liba Berry
Production Editor: Jodi Lewchuk
Cover and Interior Design: Mary Opper
Cover Image: Ray Boudreau
Author Photo: Greg Edwards
Illustrations: Dima Designs
Production Manager: Kathrine Pummell
Page Layout: Janet Zanette

1 2 3 4 5 WC 04 03 02 01 00

Printed and bound in Canada.

Visit the Prentice Hall Canada Web site! Send us your comments, browse our catalogues, and more. **www.phcanada.com**.

Prentice
Hall
Canada

A Pearson Company

dedication

to Susan, on her birthday

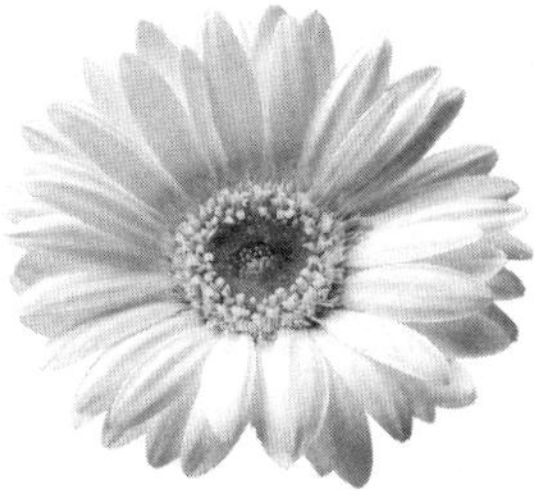

other books by M. Sara Rosenthal

The Thyroid Sourcebook

The Gynecological Sourcebook

The Pregnancy Sourcebook

The Fertility Sourcebook

The Breastfeeding Sourcebook

The Breast Sourcebook

The Gastrointestinal Sourcebook

Managing Your Diabetes

Managing Diabetes For Women

The Type 2 Diabetic Woman

The Thyroid Sourcebook for Women

Women and Sadness

Women and Depression

50 Ways To Prevent Colon Cancer

contents

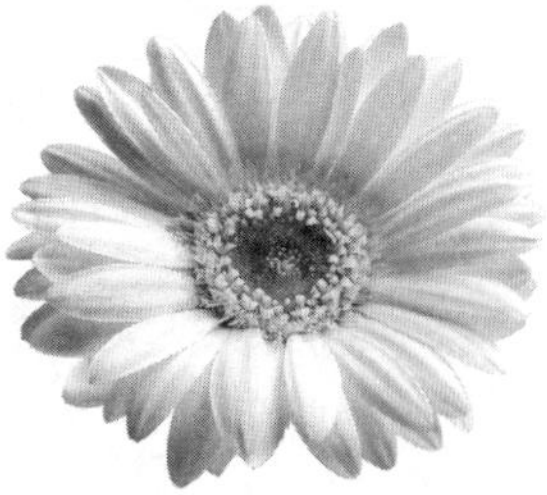

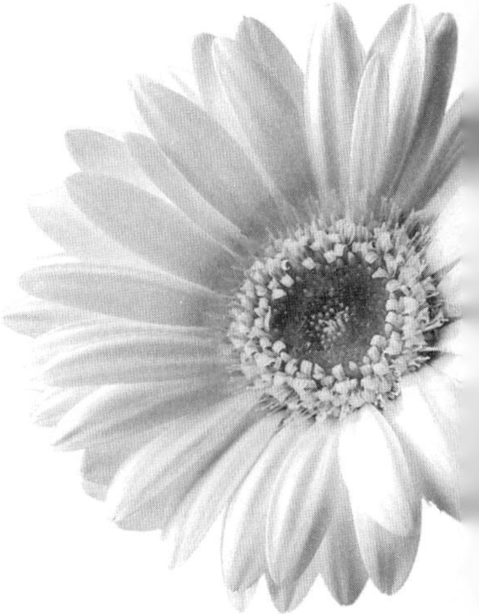

acknowledgments

I wish to thank the following people, whose expertise and dedication helped to lay so much of the groundwork for this book:

Gillian Arsenault, M.D., CC.F.P., IB.L.C., F.R.C.P.; Pamela Craig, M.D., F.A.C.S., Ph.D.; Masood Kahthamee, M.D., F.A.C.O.G.; Debra Lander, M.D., F.R.C.P.; Gary May, M.D., F.R.C.P.; James McSherry, M.B., Ch.B., F.C.F.P., FR.C.G.P., F.A.A.F.P., F.A.B.M.P.; Suzanne Pratt, M.D., FA.C.OG.; Wm Warren Rudd, M.D., F.R.C.S., F.A.C.S., colon and rectal surgeon and founder and director of the Rudd Clinic for Diseases of the Colon and Rectum (Toronto); and Robert Volpe, M.D., F.R.C.P., F.A.C.P.

William Harvey, Ph.D., L.L.B., University of Toronto Joint Centre for Bioethics, whose devotion to bioethics has inspired me, continues to support my work, and makes it possible for me to have the courage to question and challenge issues in health care and medical ethics. Irving Rootman, Ph.D., director, University of Toronto Centre for Health Promotion, continues to encourage my interest in primary prevention and health promotion issues. Helen Lenskyj, Ph.D., professor, Department of Sociology and Equity Studies, Ontario Institute for Studies in Education/University of Toronto, and Laura M. Purdy, Ph.D., professor, Department of Philosophy, University of Toronto, and bioethicist, University of Toronto, Joint Centre for Bioethics, have been central figures in my understanding the complexities of women's health issues and feminist bioethics.

Larissa Kostoff, my editorial consultant, worked very hard to make this book come into being. Liba Berry did an excellent job copy editing the book. And finally, Nicole de Montbrun, my editor, championed the project and saw how important it was for all of these health issues to come together for this unique generation of women.

What do you mean I'm going to be a GRANDMOTHER?! I was at Woodstock! I peed in a field for Chrissakes! Oh no... no, no, no... I can't be a grandmother. Grandmothers are old women who sit around telling you stories about the Depression!

— Diane Wiest in *Parenthood*

the sandwich special

As we extend our childbearing years more dramatically than ever, we find ourselves at a crossroads when it comes to relevant information for women age 50 and beyond. A significant number of women at this age have just had a child, or have a toddler at home. Books on menopause still cover issues such as empty nest syndrome when so many of us are still building the nest; or, worse, when we find ourselves trying to get our adult children to leave the nest. Studies show that far more stress is placed on women whose children won't leave, while there is a reduction in stress among women whose children have finally flown the nest. Changes in the job market mean that more young adults are extending their educations, and so more of them can't afford to leave home until they are close to 30. As they approach 50, women may also find themselves caring for their 70- or 80-something parents, which is the reason that the label "the sandwich generation" is so often applied to them.

The stress of caring for small children for women who have just started families, or started new families with second partners, the stress of caring for teens or young adult children who still haven't left home, is often combined with the stress of caring for aging parents, who may be developing, among a host of chronic ailments, Alzheimer's disease. As you cross the threshhold from parent to caregiver, you'll also be faced with the hard facts of aging: you'll need to negotiate care for your aging parents in an age where the elderly are being warehoused. There are not enough facilities to care for them, nor are the facilities that are in place well staffed. In a U.S. study, 25 percent of the women surveyed were caring for an aging parent either in their own homes or in a facility.

Many of you may also be widowed, divorced, or separated by this point in your lives, worrying about your own economic futures. And for many, no partner may have entered your life, and you may be facing angst over aging and fears of loneliness.

As all of these factors converge upon your generation, you are also being "studied." Your hearts, breasts, bones, and hormones are all being debated and discussed amongst medical experts.

In this book, I've examined the health concerns facing women of the '60s turning 50, many of whom straddle healing systems and want to know what the Western medical system offers as satisfactorily as alternative systems of healing. Much as I wanted to, I couldn't write a thousand-page encyclopedia of every conceivable health problem women face as they approach 50 and beyond. I looked at the most common health problems you're facing, as well as the health problems that were the most common concerns to *you*. For example, many of you may be much more concerned about breast cancer than colon cancer, when, in fact, colon cancer is the second leading killer cancer of both sexes next to lung cancer. Or, you may be very concerned about osteoporosis, when your risk of Type 2 diabetes is high, and carries with it many more health problems.

The goal of this book is to make you aware of what diseases may be coming down the pike as you approach menopause or perhaps are beyond it. What you need in order to protect yourself and prevent becoming debilitated by the conditions or diseases discussed in this book is all here—from West to East. Each chapter has an exhaustive What To Eat section that looks at traditional diets and nutrition as well as natural herbs and essential oils that can help strengthen various organs at risk of aging. More information about herbs and diet is provided in separate appendices. Each chapter also contains a How To Move section that combines traditional Western fitness tips with a range of postures from alternative systems of healing, such as the Ayerveda.

As mentioned above, there are health conditions that this book does not cover, such as thyroid disease, fertility issues, and urinary incontinence. In many cases I have written specific books you can consult (see Other Books on page iv). I also urge all of you to visit my Web site: **www.sarahealth.com**, and let me know what you need information on so I can build it into future editions of *Women of the '60s*. In the meantime, I hope this book offers you a chance to go beyond many of our mothers—to truly live life to the fullest for another 50 years.

foreword

Our rebellion started in the 1950s as "teenagers," a term viewed with suspicion by the powers in place at the time. At that point we were satisfied to confine our new-found individuality to our clothes and language, music and movies.

The real revolution came in the '60s as we developed a sense of our own strength and power to storm the ramparts of the establishment, the grey and nameless "they" that exerted control over every aspect of our lives from our politics to our lifestyles to our bodies. The enemy was over 30, mostly over 50. We were young, well educated, highly articulate and opinionated, and rapidly developing the philosophies and skills needed to create the new and freer world we envisioned. We were the first "Do It Yourself" generation. Publications like *The Whole Earth Catalogue* bloomed to gather our acquired knowledge into sourcebooks for the counterculture long before the Internet. We turned *The Joy of Sex* into a bestseller, and when we started to have children, we adopted Dr. Spock as our guru.

As we inevitably moved into our 30s and 40s, we turned our energy to grassroots politics, school boards, and planning councils, determined to have some control over our environment, and to make the world safer and saner for our children. We challenged the traditional male bastions of law and medicine, and forced them to address our special needs.

Now in our 50s, we have gained the luxury of concentrating on our own well-being for the first time in our lives. We are largely free of the sexual rivalry that plagued us in our 20s, and we have accomplished enough to be secure and happy in our own identities. But with that comes the realization that our bodies have changed, and probably not for the better.

Sara Rosenthal has provided us with a meticulously researched *Whole Earth Catalogue* for women's health in our 50s. She gives us the information we need to make decisions that will affect our lives well into this new century. She demystifies all the acronyms and scientific terms, and explores all the alternatives—without prejudice—in this clear and comprehensive sourcebook.

It couldn't be more timely. I only wish that our mothers had had this book.

Sylvia Tyson
–singer, songwriter, and member of the legendary '60s duo
Ian and Sylvia

one

perimenopause for hippies (or ex-hippies)

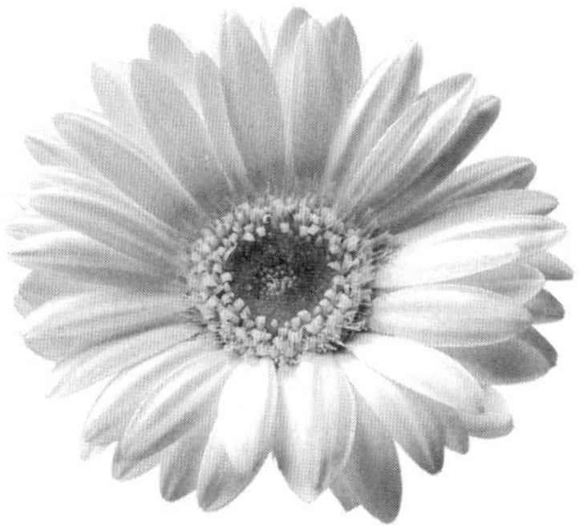

Considering the number of women who are just beginning to *really* live at 50, it seems absurd to read about menopause, doesn't it? How could you possibly relate to books about "enjoying your grandchildren" or "preparing for midlife" or "delighting in the golden years" or the dozens of other euphemisms for "hey—you're getting old!" Many of you probably have young children at home—or young lovers. Many of you are at the peak of your careers. Many of you are recently re-singled, coming out of long-term marriages or relationships. Somebody tell them to turn back the clock! You're just gettin' rollin'!

The '60s generation—a generation which defines you both indirectly and directly—has been the most powerful generation to enforce social change. In 2001, more than a million women will be between the ages of 50 and 54 in Canada alone, while almost 20 million women in the United States will be between 45 and 54—the largest number of women in that age group in all of history. Well, here's your chance to change social history once more. Nothing needs more radical social change and questioning than the positioning of menopause within our culture. And just by experiencing your own menopause, you will help to change the "change of life" for your daughters and granddaughters.

Your generation is already demedicalizing and demystifying menopause, repositioning it not as a disease but as a natural stage in life. It is up to you to take back your body, and make your own choices about how you want to live, and the quality of life you want to maintain and enjoy. This "social work" won't stop at 50, 60, 70, or even 80. We need to seriously question how our culture treats its aging and more vulnerable population. As you begin to watch your parents age, ail, and die, you will rise up and demand that the current warehousing and dismissal of our aging, vulnerable population stop. How the Western world treats its older population is unacceptable, and you're the generation that will affect the most significant social policy changes in senior health care than ever before. Why? *Because there are so many of you*. In 1994, 33 million North Americans were over 65. Now, more than 100 million North Americans are over 65. And by the year 2010, the growth rate of the older population will be three and a half times as high as that of the total population.

Native American folklore records that we are in the midst of massive earth changes that will climax around 2013, and that these earth changes will bring heat, floods, and incredible upheaval to the world's population. By then, more than 50 million women will have reached menopause and will have gone through their own heat (via hot flashes), floods (via heavy bleeding), and upheaval. Some question whether we are entering a "mass menopause" or "collective menopause." Earth changes notwithstanding, the mass menopause that will take place in the next few years will be felt. Your menopause, in many ways, is a social menopause—a time for our culture to change the way we think about aging.

This chapter gives you the facts about *perimenopause* (a term that means "around menopause"—the time when the physical signs and changes of menopause make their appearance), and both the short-term and long-term consequences of estrogen loss. At the end of this chapter, What To Eat provides information about herbal remedies, therapies, and alternatives to pharmaceutical drugs typically prescribed to women approaching menopause; and How To Move offers a range of activities, postures, and exercises that can help to offset the general discomforts of perimenopause and estrogen loss.

how menopause became a disease

If menopause is a natural stage in your life, why is it treated by the medical profession as a disease? Why is a word like "symptoms" used to describe the natural changes associated with estrogen loss? Why are you led to believe that you now have a "hormone deficiency syndrome" resulting from estrogen loss, and treated as though you are in a diseased state when you are perfectly well? The answer is simple: you live in a Western culture where *everything* is medicalized and pathologized, from womb to tomb.

It's not just menopause that is being medicalized. This trend can be seen with pregnancy and prenatal care, pediatric care (for example, millions of children are being "diagnosed" with "behaviour disorders" that in the past were considered normal), mental health (where people are put on medication for social causes of angst, anxiety, and depression), and so on. In short, *all* the normal physical processes of the human body have been pathologized by medicine.

More frequently, however, it is women's normal physical processes which are subject to the mass marketing of prevention drugs or inadequately tested therapies. In our 20s and 30s, we are sold drugs to prevent pregnancy and "regulate" our cycles. In our 30s and 40s, we are put on fertility drugs to "regulate" our cycles so we *can* get pregnant. And in our 50s and beyond, we are put on estrogen replacement drugs to "regulate" our cycles, too, and prevent health problems associated with estrogen loss. There are lots of other health conditions that sell questionable drugs to women, such as Fen/Phen for obesity (see chapter 3), and Tamoxifen for breast cancer (see chapter 4). To date, the number-one best-seller for pharmaceutical companies is hormone replacement therapy (HRT). And with the mass menopause beginning, you don't have to be a stock broker to guess that HRT "stock" stands to triple.

the lost hormone

It wasn't until the 1960s that the idea of giving estrogen to menopausal women took hold. Interestingly, this event coincided with the introduction of the birth control pill. A 1963 article by Dr. Robert Wilson, entitled "The Fate of the Nontreated Menopausal Woman: A Plea for the Maintenance of Adequate Estrogen from Puberty to the Grave," published in the *Journal of the American Geriatrics Society,* was the breakthrough article that promoted hormone replacement therapy. Wilson's article outlined the "serious consequences" of estrogen loss: heart disease, hypertension, osteoporosis, "tough, dry, scaly and inelastic skin, flabby atrophic breasts, and shrinking labia." The final blow came when Wilson stated that menopause was a "mutilation of the whole body [and that] no woman can be sure of escaping the horror of this living decay." Thus, a new "disease" was coined, and the menopause industry was born. To Wilson, estrogen loss was just like any other hormone deficiency, such as insulin in diabetes. If the lost hormone could be replaced, it *should* be replaced. This is the attitude that has prevailed.

Since Wilson, menopause apologists have surfaced in abundance, researchers who explain menopause as an accident of nature. The "apology" is an apology to women for nature's failings. You see, a woman's ovaries were supposed to work until she died; but because of a huge increase in human longevity within a short time span, there is now a gap in the natural life of a woman and the natural life of her ovaries. The message of this apology is: "It's all a big mistake; you weren't supposed to live to see menopause. It's not your fault; medicine can fix this." (In recent years the phenomenon of andropause—a deficiency of testosterone—is being sold to men as the answer to their fatigue and loss of pep in their midlife.)

Today, there are over 20 million women in North America over 50. It seems absurd to suggest that this enormous number of women are all sick and need to take medication. Yet this is the reality of our times. In essence, we are medicating huge numbers of healthy women with powerful drugs. Should doctors be doing this? Or should they sit back and allow unnecessary discomfort and suffering when it can be prevented?

Only you have the answer. If you feel physical discomfort and want your discomfort to be treated, you have that right. If you want to do everything you can to prevent the long-term complications of estrogen loss, such as osteoporosis, you have that right, too. And you have the right not to be judged by your peers for choosing to be relieved of your discomfort, or choosing preventative therapies for serious diseases associated with estrogen loss. Would your grandmother have chosen estrogen if it were offered to her? Would your grandmother have chosen to be uncomfortable when comfort was an option? Would your grandmother have chosen to experience a hip fracture or opt for information on preventing such a fate?

On the other hand, if you want to embrace the changes of your body as something nature intended, and experience your menopause as a rite of passage, so to speak, you ought not be coerced into viewing these natural changes as a disease, or into "treating" the natural rhythms and flows of your body. In many non-Western cultures, menopause is considered a powerful time for women, when they are perceived as vessels for formidable energies that flow through them. Why should you be forced to deny yourself this powerful experience? As mentioned above, you have the right not to be judged by your doctors or peers for choosing "natural menopause," just as you would not be judged for choosing natural childbirth.

Many of you will fall between these two viewpoints. You may decide to investigate diet, herbs, and simple lifestyle changes to offset your discomforts. This chapter offers a number of solutions from which to choose. Mix and match. There are no rules.

natural menopause

Your first period (menarche) and your last (menopause) have a lot in common: they are both gradual processes that you ease into. A woman doesn't suddenly wake up to find herself in menopause any more than a young girl wakes up to find herself in puberty. However, when menopause occurs *surgically*—the by-product of a bilateral oophorectomy (the surgical removal of both ovaries), ovarian failure following a hysterectomy (surgical removal of the uterus),or certain cancer therapies—it can be an extremely jarring process.

One out of three women in North America will not make it to the age of 60 with her uterus intact. These women may indeed wake up one morning to find themselves in menopause, and as a result, will suffer far more noticeable and severe signs of menopause than their natural-menopause counterparts. It is because of surgical menopause that hormonal replacement therapy (HRT) and estrogen replacement therapy (ERT or "unopposed estrogen") have become such hotly debated issues in women's health. The loss of estrogen, in particular, leads to drastic changes in the body's chemistry that trigger a more aggressive aging process. Menopause is a recent phenomenon in our society. Anywhere from 60 to 100 years ago, women simply died prior to menopause. Only in the last hundred years have women ever outlived their ovaries.

The word "menstrual" comes from the Latin word *mens*, meaning "month"; but the root word of month is "moon." The menstrual cycle actually follows the lunar calendar, not the English calendar; and in Greek, "menstruation" actually means "moon change." The word "menopause" comes from the Greek words *menos*, which means "month," and *pause*, which means "arrest"—the arrest of the menstrual cycle.

In many native cultures, menopause can be tracked by the moon. The last period, it is said, falls on the fourteenth full moon after the onset of the signs of menopause. If you track back 13 full moons on a sheet of paper after your periods have stopped, you'll find that this tracking system is pretty accurate. Apparently, by sleeping where the full moon can shine on your face when you're in the throes of menopausal changes, or by sleeping in a dark room during the full moon, and simulating moonlight with a light, your physical changes will be eased.

When menopause occurs naturally, it tends to take place anywhere between the ages of 48 and 52, but it can occur as early as your late 30s, or as late as your mid-50s. When menopause occurs before 45, it is technically considered "early menopause," but just as menarche is genetically predetermined, so is menopause. For an average woman with an unremarkable medical history, diet and level of activity will not influence the timing of her menopause. However, women who have had chemotherapy, or have been exposed to high levels of radiation, such as radiation therapy in the pelvic area for cancer treatment, may go into earlier menopause. In any event, the average age of menopause is 50 to 51.

Other triggers to an early menopause include mumps (in small groups of women, the infection causing the mumps has been known to spread to the ovaries, prematurely shutting them down); and women with specific autoimmune diseases, such as lupus or rheumatoid arthritis (some women develop antibodies to their own ovaries, which attack the ovaries).

the stages of natural menopause

Socially, the word "menopause" refers to a process, not a precise moment in the life of your menstrual cycle. Medically, the word "menopause" does indeed refer to one precise moment: the date of your last period. However, the events preceding and following menopause amount to a huge change for women both physically and socially. Physically, this process is divided into four stages:

1. *Premenopause*: although some doctors may refer to a 32-year-old woman in her child-bearing years as "premenopausal," this label is not really appropriate. The term "premenopause" ideally refers to women on the cusp of menopause. Their periods have just started to become

irregular, but they do not yet experience any classic signs of menopause, such as hot flashes or vaginal dryness. A woman in premenopause is usually in her mid to late 40s. If your doctor tells you that you're premenopausal, you might want to ask how this term is being used.

2. *Perimenopause:* this term refers to women who are in the thick of menopause—their cycles are wildly erratic, they are experiencing hot flashes and vaginal dryness. This label applies for about four years, covering the first two years prior to the official last period to the next two years following the last menstrual period. Women who are perimenopausal will be in the age groups discussed above, averaging to about 51.
3. *Menopause:* this term refers to your final menstrual period. You will not be able to pinpoint your final period until you've been completely free from periods for one year. Then you count back to the last period you charted, and *that* date is the date of your menopause. (Note: after more than one year of no menstrual periods, any vaginal bleeding is considered abnormal.)
4. *Postmenopause:* this term refers to the last third of most women's lives, ranging from women who have been free of menstrual periods for at least four years to women celebrating their hundredth birthday. In other words, once you're past menopause, you'll be referred to as postmenopausal for the rest of your life. Sometimes, the terms "postmenopausal" and "perimenopausal" are used interchangeably, but this is technically inaccurate.

Used in a social context, however, nobody really bothers to break down menopause as precisely. When you see the word "menopausal" in a magazine article, you are seeing what's become acceptable medical slang, referring to women who are premenopausal and perimenopausal—a time frame that includes the actual menopause. When you see the word "postmenopausal" in a magazine article, you are seeing another expression of accepted medical slang, which includes women who are in perimenopause and "official" postmenopause.

determining premenopause or perimenopause

When you begin to notice the signs of menopause, either you'll suspect the approach of menopause on your own, or your doctor will put two and two together when you report your "bizarre symptoms."

There are two very simple, painless tests that will accurately determine what's going on, and what stage of menopause you're in. Your FSH (follicle stimulating hormone) levels will dramatically rise as your ovaries begin to shut down (see below); these levels are easily checked in one blood test. In addition, your vaginal walls will thin, and the cells lining the vagina will not contain as much estrogen. Your doctor will simply do a Pap-like smear on your vaginal walls, and then analyze the smear to check for vaginal atrophy, the thinning and drying out of your vagina.

In addition, you need to keep track of your menstrual periods and chart them as they become irregular. Your menstrual pattern will be an additional clue to your doctor about whether you are pre- or perimenopausal.

signs of natural menopause

In the past, a long list of psychiatric symptoms have been attributed to the "change of life," but medically there are three classic short-term signs of menopause: erratic menstrual periods, hot flashes, and vaginal dryness. All three signs are caused by a decrease in estrogen. The emotional signs of menopause, such as irritability, mood swings, melancholy, and so on are actually caused by a rise in FSH, the hormone that promotes the formation of ova. As the cycle changes and the ovaries' egg supply dwindles, FSH is secreted in very high amounts and reach a lifetime peak—as much as 15 times higher; it's the body's way of trying to jump-start the ovarian engine. This is why the urine of menopausal women is used to produce human menopausal gonadotropin (HMG), the potent fertility drug that consists of pure FSH.

Every woman entering menopause will experience a change in her menstrual cycle. However, not all women will experience hot flashes or even notice vaginal changes. This is particularly true if a woman is overweight. Estrogen is stored in fat cells, which is why overweight women also tend to be more at risk for estrogen-dependent cancers such as breast cancer and ovarian cancer. The fat cells convert fat into estrogen, creating a type of estrogen reserve that the body will use during menopause, which can reduce the severity of estrogen loss.

erratic menstrual periods

Every woman will begin to experience an irregular cycle before her last period. Cycles may become longer or shorter with long bouts of amennorhea. There will also be flow changes; periods may suddenly become light and scanty, or very heavy and crampy. The heavy bleeding occurs because of a sudden drop in progesterone levels (this is why all women get their periods). But when progesterone levels are higher than normal for a premenopausal women, the uterine lining just keeps growing thicker. Then, when you do bleed, it just floods and gushes. It's not unusual to bleed heavily for as long as 10–14 days. You will lose iron when you bleed this heavily. See the What To Eat section for iron-rich herbs and foods.

keeping your cool about hot flashes

Roughly 85 per cent of all pre- and perimenopausal women experience what's known as hot flashes. Eastern cultures view a hot flash as a release of cosmic electricity, known as kundalini energies, which not only rewires your individual nervous system, but also gives you healing energies for your entire community. The intensity of your hot flash can be compared to the intensity felt during anger, orgasm, or even enlightenment, which all involve kundalini energies, too.

Hot flashes can begin when periods are either still regular, or have just started to become irregular; and usually stop between one to two years after your final menstrual period. A hot flash can feel different for each woman. Some women experience a feeling of warmth in their face and upper body; some experience hot flashes as a simultaneous sweating with chills. Some women feel anxious, tense, dizzy, or nauseous just before the hot flash; some feel tingling in their fingers or heart palpitations just before. Some women experience their hot flashes during the day; others experience them at night, and may wake up so wet from perspiration that they need to change their bedsheets and nightclothes.

Although hot flashes are harmless in terms of health risks, they are disquieting and stressful. Yet certain groups of women will experience more severe hot flashes than others: women who are in surgical menopause; women who are thin—when there's less fat on the body to store estrogen reserves, physical changes associated with estrogen loss are more severe; and women who don't sweat easily—an ability to sweat makes extreme temperatures easier to tolerate.

Nobody really understands what causes a hot flash, but researchers believe that it has to do with mixed signals from the hypothalamus, the region of the brain that controls both body temperature and sex hormones.

Normally, when the body is too warm, the hypothalamus sends a chemical message to the heart to cool off the body by pumping more blood, causing the blood vessels under the skin to dilate, which makes you perspire. During menopause, however, it's believed that the hypothalamus gets confused and sends this cooling-off signal at the wrong times.

A hot flash is not the same as being overheated. Although the skin temperature often rises between 4 to 8 degrees Fahrenheit, the internal body temperature drops, creating this odd sensation. Why does the hypothalamus get so confused? Decreasing levels of estrogen. We know this because when synthetic estrogen is given to replace natural estrogen in the body, hot flashes disappear. Some researchers believe that a decrease in luteinizing hormone (LH), the hormone that stimulates ovulation, is also a key factor, and a variety of other hormones that influence body temperature are being looked at as well.

Just as you must chart your periods when your cycles become irregular, it's also important to chart your hot flashes. Record when the flashes occur and how long they last, and number their intensity from 1 to 10. This will help you determine a pattern for the flashes, and allow you to prepare for them in advance, which will reduce the stress involved in the flashes to begin with. It's also crucial to report your hot flashes to your doctor, just as you would any changes in your cycle. Hot flashes can also indicate other health problems, such as circulatory problems.

what can I do about my hot flashes?

Short of taking ERT or HRT, you can lessen the discomfort of hot flashes by adjusting your lifestyle to cope with them. The more comfortable you are, the less intense your flashes will feel. Once you establish a pattern by charting them, try some of the following around the time of day your flashes occur:

- Avoid wearing clothing made of synthetic fibres, such as polyester because it traps perspiration.
- Use only 100 per cent cotton bedding if you have night sweats.
- Avoid wearing clothing with high necks and long sleeves.
- Dress in layers.
- Keep cold drinks handy.
- Quit smoking. Smoking constricts blood vessels and can intensify and prolong a flash.

- Avoid consuming trigger foods such as caffeine, alcohol, spicy foods, sugars, and eating large meals. Substitute herbal teas for coffee or regular tea.
- Discuss the benefits of taking vitamin E supplements with your doctor. Evidence suggests that vitamin E is essential for proper circulation and the production of sex hormones.
- Exercise to improve your circulation. (See How to Move.)
- Reduce your exposure to the sun. Sunburn aggravates hot flashes because burnt skin cannot regulate heat as effectively.

vaginal changes

Estrogen loss will also cause vaginal changes. Since it is the production of estrogen that causes the vagina to continuously stay moist and elastic through its natural secretions, the loss of estrogen will cause the vagina to become drier, thinner, and less elastic. This may also cause the vagina to shrink slightly in width and length. In addition, the reduction in vaginal secretions causes the vagina to be less acidic. This can put you at risk for more vaginal infections. As a result of these vaginal changes, you'll notice a change in your sexual activity. Your vagina may take longer to become lubricated, or you may have to depend on lubricants to have comfortable intercourse.

Estrogen loss can affect other parts of your sex life as well. Your libido may actually increase because testosterone levels can rise when estrogen levels drop. (Generally, your levels of testosterone will either stay the same or increase.) However, women who do experience an increase in sexual desire will also be frustrated that their vaginas are not accommodating their needs. First, there is the lubrication problem: more stimulation is required to lubricate the vagina naturally. Second, a decrease in estrogen means that less blood flows to the vagina and clitoris, which means that orgasm may be more difficult to achieve or may not last as long as it normally has in the past. Third, estrogen loss causes less blood to flow to the breasts, which makes them less sensitive. Normally, estrogen causes blood to flow into the breasts during arousal, which makes the nipples more erect, sensitive, and responsive. And finally, since the vagina shrinks as estrogen decreases, it doesn't expand as much during intercourse, which may make intercourse less comfortable, particularly since it is less lubricated.

surgical menopause

Surgical menopause is the result of a bilateral oophorectomy, the removal of both ovaries before natural menopause. Surgical menopause can also be the result of ovarian failure following a hysterectomy or following cancer therapy, such as chemotherapy or radiation treatments. A bilateral oophorectomy is often done in conjunction with a hysterectomy, or sometimes as a single procedure, when ovarian cancer is suspected, for example. In this section, I refer to menopause "symptoms" instead of signs or changes, because menopause, in this case, is medically induced, rather than a natural occurrence.

bilateral oophorectomy

If you've had your ovaries removed after menopause, you won't be in surgical menopause. You won't feel any hormonal differences in your body, although you may experience some structural problems. If you've had your ovaries removed before you've reached natural menopause, you'll wake up from your surgery in postmenopause. Once the ovaries are removed, your body immediately stops producing estrogen and progesterone. Your FSH will skyrocket in an attempt to make contact with ovaries that no longer exist.

Unlike women who go through menopause naturally, women wake up after a bilateral oophorectomy in immediate estrogen "withdrawal." It's that sudden: one day you have a normal menstrual cycle, the next, you have none whatsoever. This can cause you to become understandably more depressed, but you'll also feel the physical symptoms of estrogen loss far more intensely than a woman in natural menopause. That means that your vagina will be extremely dry, your hot flashes will feel like sudden violent heat waves that will be very disturbing to your system, and of course, your periods will cease altogether, instead of tapering off naturally.

The menstrual period that you had prior to your surgery will have been your last, so you won't even experience pre- or perimenopause, just postmenopause. That means that you'll need to begin estrogen replacement therapy immediately following surgery to prevent these sudden symptoms of menopause. As discussed in greater detail below, if you no longer have your uterus, you'll be put on estrogen only, or unopposed estrogen. If you still have your uterus, you'll be placed on estrogen and progesterone hormone replacement therapy, for the reasons below. Any short-term menopausal symptoms will be alleviated by HRT/ERT. Prior to your going on HRT/ERT, your doctor will perform a vaginal smear and a blood test to detect your FSH levels, which will indicate how much estrogen you need. Dosages will vary from woman to woman, so don't compare notes with your friends and wonder why she's taking only X amount when you're taking Y amount.

if you've just had one ovary removed...

If the blood supply leading to your ovary was not damaged during surgery, you should still be able to produce enough estrogen for your body. If you begin to go into ovarian failure, the symptoms will depend on how fast the ovary is failing; you may experience symptoms more akin to natural menopause, or you may experience sudden symptoms, mirroring the surgical menopause experience.

ovarian failure resulting from cancer therapy

Chemotherapy and radiation treatments that involve the pelvic area may throw your ovaries into menopause. As above, you may experience a more gradual menopausal process, or you may be overwhelmed by sudden symptoms of menopause. This depends on what kind of therapy you've received and the speed at which your ovaries are failing. Before you undergo cancer treatment, discuss with your doctor how the treatments will affect your ovaries, and what menopausal symptoms you can expect.

long-term effects of estrogen loss: postmenopausal changes

The long-term effects of estrogen loss have to do with the traditional signs of aging. One of the key reasons that women will choose HRT or ERT is to slow down or even reverse these changes. It's important to keep in mind that the long-term effects of estrogen loss will not immediately set in after menopause. These changes are subtle, and happen over several years. Even women who experience severe menopausal changes will not wake up to find that they've suddenly aged overnight; these changes occur gradually whether you experience surgical *or* natural menopause.

skin changes

As estrogen decreases, skin, like the vagina, tends to lose elasticity; it too becomes thinner because it is no longer able to retain as much water. Sweat and oil glands also produce less moisture, which is what causes the skin to gradually dry, wrinkle, and sag.

Good moisturizers and skin care will certainly help to keep your skin more elastic, but there is one known factor that aggravates and speeds up your skin's natural aging process, damaging the skin even more: the sun.

If you cut down your sun exposure, you can dramatically reduce visible aging of your skin. Period. The bad news is that much of the sun's damage on skin is cumulative from many years of exposure. In fact, many researchers believe that when it comes to visible signs of aging, estrogen loss is only a small factor. For example, it's known that ultraviolet rays (UV) break down collagen and elastin fibres in the skin, which cause it to break down and sag. Exposure to UV rays is also what puts us at risk for skin cancer, the most notorious of which is melanoma, one of the most aggressive and malignant of all cancers.

Other sun-related skin problems traditionally linked to estrogen loss are "liver spots"—light brown or tan splotches that develop on the face, neck, and hands as we age. These spots have nothing to do with the liver; they are sun spots and are caused by sun exposure. In fact, they are sometimes the result of HRT, known in this case as *hyperpigmentation*.

Currently, dermatologists are recommending sunblocks with a minimum of SPF 15. In fact, sun damage is so widespread in our population that today sunblock is usually part the daily cosmetic routine of all North American women; many women apply it as regularly as a daily moisturizer.

hormone replacement therapy (HRT)

The average North American woman will live until age 78, meaning that she will live one-third of her life after her menopause. Since women are more prone to heart disease as a result of estrogen loss after menopause, discuss with your doctor whether hormone replacement therapy is an option for you after menopause. The Women's Health Initiative (WHI) is currently studying 25,000 postmenopausal women. The results of this study, anticipated by 2003, are expected to present more concrete facts regarding the benefits of HRT on postmenopausal women with a myriad of other health problems.

Many women, of course, will also be concerned about their risk of breast cancer. Taking estrogen can stimulate or trigger the growth of an estrogen-dependent breast cancer cell, that is, a breast cancer cell that feeds, or thrives on, the hormone estrogen. Studies show that these types of cancers are far more treatable than other kinds of breast cancers. More women, however, die from heart attacks than breast cancer after menopause. The risk of dying from a heart attack may increase if you suffered damage to your heart as a result of prolonged and untreated hyper or hypothryoidism. So, preventing heart disease, as well as fractures from osteoporosis, is considered to be a benefit for postmenopausal women. Nevertheless, you have some thinking to do if you're considering hormone replacement therapy. Here are the facts you need in order to make a more informed choice.

what is HRT?

Hormone replacement therapy (HRT) refers to the hormones estrogen *and* progesterone; the progesterone is given to women after menopause who still have a uterus to prevent the uterine lining from overgrowing and becoming cancerous. Estrogen replacement therapy (ERT) refers to estrogen only, which is given to women after surgical menopause who no longer have a uterus. Both HRT and ERT are designed to replace the estrogen lost after menopause, and hence: prevent or even reverse the long-term consequences of estrogen loss (osteoporosis, skin changes, vaginal thinning and dryness, and many other ailments); and treat the short-term discomforts of menopause such as hot flashes and vaginal dryness.

Therefore, you have the choice of taking HRT or ERT as either a short-term therapy or a long-term therapy. However, there are also some risks involved with HRT and ERT that you'll need to weigh against the benefits.

the benefits

What exactly is estrogen responsible for in our bodies? In addition to protecting our bones and maintaining our reproductive organs, estrogen also helps to maintain appropriate levels of high-density lipoproteins (HDL), which keeps our arteries clear of plaque, preventing them from clogging and causing heart attacks and strokes. By raising HDL, known as the "good" cholesterol, the "bad" cholesterol, the low-density lipoproteins (LDL) that cause fatty substances to collect in the arteries (causing arteriosclerosis, or hardening of the arteries) drop.

Estrogen also helps protect us from rheumatoid arthritis. It's our ovaries, of course that make estrogen, but other sources of estrogen come from the hormones androstenedione and testosterone, which are converted by our tissues into a form of estrogen called *estrone*, a weaker form of estrogen than the kind our ovaries produce. Obese women have estrone in greater amounts. Although this may prevent any severe menopausal changes, estrone is not considered a potent enough form of estrogen to protect against osteoporosis or heart disease.

Thirty years ago, all women, regardless of whether they still had a uterus, were placed on pure estrogen hormone without any progesterone. This is known as unopposed estrogen therapy because in a natural cycle the progesterone opposes the estrogen and counterbalances high estrogen levels, preventing the body from becoming estrogen toxic at far higher dosages than what's given today. This created several problems. First, women experienced side effects similar to those experienced on early oral contraceptives: nausea, dizziness, bloating, and so on. Second, women who went into menopause naturally tended to develop endometrial hyperplasia (overgrowth of the uterine lining) which often became uterine cancer. Finally, both surgical and natural menopause recipients of unopposed estrogen therapy were considered at higher risk of developing estrogen-dependent cancers.

Today, all women who have gone through menopause naturally, who decide to go on HRT, will be given both estrogen and progesterone. The progesterone triggers the uterine lining to shed regularly, which prevents endometrial hyperplasia, which is what predisposes women who are on unopposed estrogen (those with a uterus, taking only estrogen) to develop uterine cancer. Estrogen and progesterone together also mirror the normal menstrual cycle, and help prevent the side effects normally felt with solo estrogen. Current ERT doses are much lower than they were in the past; current HRT doses are about ten times lower than the average combination oral contraceptive (OC).

If you're in surgical menopause you won't need any progesterone because you're not at risk for endometrial hyperplasia anymore. However, because your menopausal changes will be more severe, your need for estrogen may be greater. But again, since current estrogen doses are so much lower, you'll likely not experience any short-term side effects from the estrogen.

what to expect in the short term

Generally, HRT/ERT will begin to relieve the discomforts associated with estrogen loss within days of starting the therapy. Your hot flashes will disappear, your vagina will become moist again and will lubricate on its own during sex, and the acidic environment of your vagina will be restored, preventing yeast and other vaginal infections from plaguing you. However, if you change your mind and go off the therapy, your discomfort will return in a far more severe form.

what to expect in the long term

Your HDL levels will be maintained, and you won't experience any severe bone loss, which can put you at risk for fractures and breakages. However, research shows that HRT is more effective than ERT in preventing osteoporosis (see chapter 6).

As for heart disease, see chapter 2 for a detailed discussion.

the risks

The risk that we hear about most regarding the estrogen issue is uterine cancer. Today, this is no longer a risk. In the past, unopposed estrogen was given both to women who still had a uterus and women without one. Of course, if you don't have a uterus, there is no risk of uterine cancer. But what about the women who had one? Well, a funny thing happened: doctors forgot about the uterus, ignoring that the female body is very smart. When it detects estrogen, it says: "Oh, look—estrogen again! Better start preparing the endometrium for a baby!" And guess what? There's no progesterone to trigger the lining to shed, and certainly no baby, so the lining just keeps growing until you wind up with endometrial hyperplasia, and eventually, uterine cancer. When the uterine cancer rate began to increase in uterus "owners" on unopposed estrogen, the medical community realized its mistake, remembered the uterus and the importance of progesterone, and today, will not administer unopposed estrogen to any woman with a uterus.

being a slave to the medical system

An obvious, but underreported risk of HRT is that it forces you into another continuous cycle of constant doctor visits and tests. Each time you go to your doctor, you risk some sort of invasive procedure or referral for invasive tests.

For example, women on HRT are more likely to be prescribed the following tests or medications:

- Blood tests for hormone levels
- Diuretics for fluid retention
- Ponstan, aspirin, or other analgesics for uterine cramps
- Endometrial biopsies to check the endometrium
- D & C (dilation and curettage) for bleeding
- Blood pressure tests
- Blood tests for cholesterol levels
- Baseline mammograms before starting therapy and regular mammograms thereafter
- Visits for repeat prescriptions of hormones at least every six months

Women who are not on HRT are not burdened by as many tests, visits, and other medical procedures. Do these increased visits to the doctor save lives because they offer early detection of many serious diseases? Critics of HRT argue that women are paying a higher price for their dependency on the medical system, and are burdened with too much monitoring and early detection.

the forms of HRT and ERT

You can take estrogen in a number of ways. The most common estrogen product uses a synthesis of various estrogens that are derived from the urine of pregnant mares. That way, the estrogen mimics nature more accurately. Estrogen replacement comes in either pills, transdermal patches, or vaginal creams. Other common, synthetic forms of estrogen include micronized estradiol, ethinyl estradiol, esterified estrogen, and quinestrol.

As a short-term therapy, you may only need the vaginal cream to help with vaginal dryness or bladder problems. As a long-term therapy, you'll need the pill form if you want to protect yourself from heart disease. Premarin comes under a variety of brand names, each just as good as the other. Estrogen can also be worn. In this case, it's placed in a small plastic patch which is about the size of a silver dollar, worn on the abdomen, thighs, or buttocks, and changed twice weekly.

When estrogen is taken in patch or cream form, it goes directly to the bloodstream, bypassing the liver, and hence does not affect HDL, or protect against heart disease. Some women also have an allergic reaction to the skin patch and get a rash. If you're one of them, investigate taking the estrogen in other forms.

Finally, you can also have estrogen injected. Each shot lasts between 3–6 weeks, but this is expensive and inconvenient because the dosages aren't as flexible with shots. Estrogen gel containing estradiol is now being used in some parts of the world, though it is not yet available in North America. The gel is spread over a wide area of the abdomen every second day. The problem women have encountered with this method is a variation in levels of absorption each time the gel is applied.

Even more controversial are the pellets or implants containing estradiol inserted under the skin of the abdomen or buttock under local anesthetic. Subcutaneous implants are not yet available in North America, primarily because they are difficult to remove or halt if a woman experiences complications.

Women react differently to Premarin or other synthetic forms of estrogen; some do better than others on different chemical recipes. So, if you don't do well on Premarin, for example, see if estradiol is better for you, or vice versa. Don't just give up and go off HRT or ERT altogether; explore all the estrogen possibilities. Dosages are discussed below.

progesterone

Synthetic progestins, a family of progesterone drugs that include natural progesterone, are norethridone or norethindrone acetate. Natural progestin is medroxyprogesterone.

Progestins are taken in separate tablets along with estrogen. Together, the estrogen and progestin you take is called HRT. HRT can be administered two ways: cyclically or continuously.

Taking HRT cyclically is very similar to taking an oral contraceptive because the hormones more closely mirror a natural cycle. The first day you start is considered day 1 of your mock cycle. You take estrogen from day 1–25; you then add the progesterone from day 14–25. Then you stop all pills and bleed for two or three days, just as you would on a combination oral contraceptive. This vaginal bleeding is called withdrawal bleeding, which is lighter and shorter than a normal menstrual period, lasting only two or three days, like a period on a combination OC. In fact, if the bleeding is heavy or prolonged for some reason, this is a warning that something's not right, and you should get it checked.

In addition, you may experience breakthrough bleeding—spotting during the first three weeks after you begin HRT. This kind of bleeding is, again, similar to what happens on a combination OC. It usually goes away after a few months, but report it to your doctor anyway. You may need to switch to a lower dose of estrogen or take a higher dose of progestin. Once your mini-period of withdrawal bleeding is finished, you simply start the cycle again. Many women can't tolerate cyclical HRT because they feel as though they should be rid of their periods by now, and not have to deal with pads and tampons ever again. However, it is believed that cyclical HRT offers slightly better heart protection.

When HRT is taken continuously, you take one estrogen pill and one progestin pill each day. When you do it this way, the progesterone counteracts the estrogen; no uterine lining is built up, so there's no withdrawal bleeding that needs to happen.

the appropriate dosages

Every woman requires a different dosage of estrogen and progestin. But you will always be placed on the lowest possible dosage of either one, and may have the dosage increased gradually if necessary. If your estrogen dosage is too high, you'll experience side effects similar to those seen with oral contraceptives: headaches, bloating, and so on.

So before you determine how much estrogen you'll need, it's crucial to determine how much your body is still producing; the amount depends on your weight, estrogen loss discomforts, and a hundred other things.

common side effects

If you're taking cyclical progestins with your estrogen because you still have your uterus, bleeding is *not* a side effect! The whole point of adding progestin to your estrogen is to trigger withdrawal bleeding, and get your uterine lining routinely shed. However, if you're taking continuous progestins with your estrogen, bleeding is not the norm, and should be checked into.

Common side effects of estrogen therapy will be fluid retention, because estrogen will decrease the amount of salt and water excreted by the kidneys, which is retained by the legs, breasts, and feet, which can swell. Because of the fluid retention, you may weigh more, but you might also gain weight. Nausea is another common side effect, also seen with OCs. You might experience this during the first two or three months of your therapy, and it should disappear on its own. Some women find that taking their dosages at night (for pills) may remedy this. Decreasing the dosage is also an option.

Other side effects of estrogen therapy include: headaches, skin colour changes, called *melasma*, on the face, excessive cervical mucus secretion, liquid secretion from the breasts (consult your doctor), change in curvature of the cornea, jaundice, loss of scalp hair, and itchiness. Again, these side effects vary and depend on the brand you're taking, the dosage, your medical history, and so on.

are you an HRT or ERT candidate?

As mentioned above, HRT or ERT is not for everyone. Some women make better candidates than others. Here's a guide that can help you make the decision:

- Do you suffer from severe hot flashes that don't respond to natural remedies? (see page 10)
- Are your vaginal changes causing painful intercourse, urinary tract infections (UTIs), or vaginitis, which does not respond to natural remedies or sexual lubricants?
- Are you in a high-risk category for endometrial cancer? If so, taking progestin to trigger withdrawal bleeding will lower your risk.
- Are you in a high-risk group for heart attacks or strokes? If so, ERT or HRT will lower your risk.
- Are you in a high-risk group for developing osteoporosis? Again, ERT or HRT will lower your risk. (But so will exercise and a high-calcium diet.)

women who shouldn't be on ERT or HRT

- Women with (a history of) endometrial cancer should not be on unopposed estrogen ERT. Again, if you still have a uterus, you'll be placed on HRT (estrogen and progesterone), which lowers your cancer risk anyway.
- Women with breast cancer. This is in debate. (See below)
- Women who have had a stroke.
- Women who have a blood-clotting disorder.
- Women with undiagnosed vaginal bleeding.
- Women with liver dysfunction. You can be on the estrogen patch or vaginal cream to relieve your menopausal discomforts, but you shouldn't take any pills orally.

women who may benefit more from HRT/ERT

Discuss with your doctor whether you're a candidate for HRT, given its protective effects against osteoporosis and heart disease. However, you may need to think twice if you have the following other conditions: sickle cell disease; high blood pressure (hypertension); migraines; uterine fibroids; a history of benign breast conditions such as cysts or fibroadenomas; endometriosis; seizures; gallbladder disease; a family history of breast cancer; a past or current history of smoking.

concerns about breast cancer

Postmenopausal breast cancer is considered to be epidemic among women over 50. The reasons for this are discussed in chapter 4. Women at risk for heart disease (see chapter 2), a disease from which they are two to three times more likely to suffer than the average woman, will probably be told that they should consider HRT to reduce their risk. Therefore, you may be concerned about breast cancer risk and HRT.

It's still not clear whether HRT increases your risk of breast cancer, but there's actually more consensus in the medical research community over this issue than many others. That's because the incidence of breast cancer in Western nations dramatically rises anyway after menopause, whether you're on HRT or not. So it's not clear whether HRT really contributes to this increase. The current thinking seems to be that if you're on HRT there's a slight increased risk of developing breast cancer. But if you do develop it, it's apparently a very treatable type of cancer that's estrogen-receptor positive, which means that your risk of dying from breast cancer is decreased.

If you add up all the data, you may want to rethink HRT if your risk of breast cancer is significant (see chapter 4), or if the risk of breast cancer significantly outweighs your risk of heart disease. For the record, heart disease kills more women than breast cancer, and HRT can definitely lower your cholesterol levels, lower your risk of heart disease, and your risk of dying from heart disease. Furthermore, if you are at greater risk for osteoporosis, HRT can help to stop bone loss. In fact, if started in the first few years after menopause, HRT will even increase bone mass. Remember, hip and spinal fractures can be very debilitating, often life-threatening, and can truly affect quality of life (See chapter 6).

natural hormone replacement therapy (NHRT)

Many of you may have heard the media hype surrounding natural hormone replacement therapy (NHRT), which includes natural progesterone, versus conventional hormone replacement therapy. The difference is akin to breast milk and formula for a baby.

NHRT is a combination of human estrogens and natural human progesterone. HRT, on the other hand, is a factory-made estrogen, much of which is derived from horse estrogen, and a factory-made progesterone, called progestin. Studies show that the symptoms of menopause are better controlled with NHRT with fewer side effects. Studies also show that the benefits of HRT—protection from heart disease and osteoporosis—are more dramatic and pronounced using NHRT.

what NHRT contains

When you go on NHRT, you're getting about 60–80 per cent estriol; 10–20 per cent estrone, and 10–20 per cent estradiol, as well as natural human progesterone, and DHEA (dehydroepiandrosterone), a natural androgen which turns into a natural testosterone in the body, something all women need in order to maintain their sex drive. On HRT, you're getting 75–80 per cent estrone, 6–15 per cent equilin, a horse-derived estrogen, and about 5–19 per cent estradiol, as well as progestin, a factory-made progesterone, and, sometimes, anabolic steroids if your libido needs a boost.

The bottom line is that women do better with human hormones than with animal-derived hormones, just as infants do better on human milk than cow's milk. However, as you can see from the range of concentrations of various natural estrogens, it may take a while for you to find just the right dose of each kind of natural estrogen and progesterone, so you have to work with your doctor and experiment until you get it right.

There is a perception that NHRT is perfect the first time you take it, and many women have to tinker with their "triple estrogens" before they find the right combination for them. A typical prescription for NHRT is often 10 per cent estrone, 10 per cent estradiol, and 80 per cent estriol, mixed with about 25–30 mg of natural progesterone after menopause, and 10–30 mg DHEA, which should, but doesn't always, convert into necessary amounts of testosterone. If it doesn't, you may need to add a steroid to the mix of natural hormones if your libido is very low, which can be debilitating.

where do you find NHRT?

Books and articles about NHRT can mislead you into thinking that they are available everywhere. This is not so. You can't just walk into a health food store and buy natural estrogens or progesterones. They need to be prescribed by a doctor, although the doctor need not be an M.D.; several naturopathic doctors prescribe them, too.

A pharmacist has to prepare a doctor's prescription for NHRT from scratch. This individual is known as a compounding pharmacist. Not all pharmacies are compounding pharmacies, so ask your doctor or pharmacist where to get a prescription prepared. You can also call the International Academy of Compounding Pharmacists (IACP) or the Professional Compounding Centers of America, Inc. (PCCA) for the nearest compounding pharmacist in your area. Several Canadian compounding pharmacists are members of either or both organizations. You can reach the PCCA at 800-331-2498 or at **www.compassnet.com/~iacp/**.

phytoestrogens: the HRT alternative

If you are uncomfortable with the idea of taking any kind of hormone replacement therapy, you may wish to consider the therapeutic benefits of phytoestrogens, or plant estrogens.

Phytoestrogens contain a multitude of chemicals, including estrogenic substances. Although phytoestrogens have been used in Asian cultures for centuries to treat hot flashes, they're just beginning to catch on in the West. The first controlled trial began in 1996 at Columbia-Presbyterian Medical Center in New York.

Many food sources, such as tofu and soy, contain such high concentrations of phytoestrogens, scientists believe it may account for the incredible lack of menopausal discomforts in Japan, which has a soy-heavy diet. Blood levels of phytoestrogens are 10 to 40 times higher in Japanese women than in their Western counterparts, but Japanese women report hot flashes about one-sixth as often as Western women. Even the average vegetarian would not consume nearly as much soy as the average Japanese woman.

More interesting, plant hormones not only help prevent menopausal discomforts, they may also protect you from breast cancer. Breast cancer rates are dramatically lower in Japan than in the United States, but other factors might account for this, such as child-bearing habits and low-fat diets. After menopause, high-fat diets can increase your risk of heart attack and stroke, no matter how much estrogen you take. Meanwhile, engaging in bad habits, such as drinking coffee and alcohol, and smoking, can all increase your risk of osteoporosis. Most doctors will tell you to go ahead and add as much soy as you want to your diet. It may well help; and it certainly can't hurt. Soy has most recently been declared a heart healthy food (see chapter 2). Moreover, many women treat their discomforts with herbs, outlined in the What To Eat section at the end of this chapter.

what are the drawbacks?

The problem with phytoestrogens is that they are plant hormones, not human hormones, which means that they will not solve the problem of rising FSH and LH levels, the gonadotropins that kick-start the ovaries. However, some plants do encourage estrogen production, and some do contain flavonoids, which are estrogen-like.

Plant hormones can be converted to human hormones in a laboratory. What plant hormones do is to provide you with hormonal building blocks rather than hormones themselves, which, in theory, can allow you to create the amounts, and combinations, of hormones you need for your unique menopausal journey.

Phytoestrogens can be taken orally or even in creams, which can be applied to parts of your body. Creams are quasi-natural, however, because the plant hormones they contain are modified in a lab.

One good question many women ask is whether phytoestrogens carry the same risks as HRT. The answer is that because plant-based hormones contain chemicals that are similar, but not identical, to your natural estrogen, you may still suffer from discomfort associated with estrogen loss in spite of your dedication to ingesting plant hormones. Moreover, it is possible to have allergic reactions to a variety of herbs. It's also important to note that because herbal products are not regulated, there is a danger of misuse, overuse, or use of poor-quality merchandise.

what to eat

This section gives you plenty of ideas if you're wondering about herbal remedies, nourishing and tonifying herbs during perimenopause and after menopause. The variety in this section is meant to give you choices, not to insist that you try everything. Have fun. You may wish to start an herbal group, where you and some of your friends compare notes with what works best. Also, see the appendices and Tables 1.1 and 1.2 for more ideas.

HOW TO HAVE SAFE HERBS

1. Buy herbs that are labelled with the botanical name specific to only one plant. For example, "sage" can refer to at least five plants in five different areas, but *Salvia officinalis* means garden sage only.
2. Introduce yourself to one herb at a time, and try to learn all you can about your "new herb." That means experimenting: Does it work best at different times of day, or with certain foods or other herbs you know well?
3. Herbs can be "tonic" (maintenance herbs) or "active" (sedating or stimulating). Tonic herbs include: birch, black cohosh, blackstrap molasses, chaste tree, dandelion, Dong Quai/Dang Gui, echinacea, false unicorn, ginseng, hawthorn, horsetail, lady's mantle, motherwort, peony, sarsaparilla, spikenard, wild yam, and yellow dock. "Active" herbs include: catnip, cinnamon, ginger, hops, licorice, myrrh, passion flower, poplar, primrose, sage, skullcap, uva ursi, valerian, vervain, willow, and wintergreen.
4. Herbs can also be toxic in high quantities. Toxic herbs include: cayenne, cotton root, goldenseal, liferoot, poke root, rue, sweet clover (Melilot), and wormseed.

for irregular menstrual periods

estrogen herbs

The following herbs help promote estrogen production, stabilize infrequent periods, and may reduce the severity of estrogen-loss discomforts:

- Alfalfa and red clover flowers/leaves
- Black cohosh roots
- Hops (female flowers)
- Licorice roots
- Sage leaves
- Sweet briar hips or leaf buds
- Pomegranate seeds
- Any herb containing flavonoids

progesterone herbs

The following herbs help promote progesterone production and help stabilize too-frequent periods:

- Chaste tree/vitex berries
- Sarsaparilla roots
- Wild yam roots
- Yarrow flowers and leaves

phytoestrogens

The following are plant estrogens, which may help with a myriad of menopausal discomforts:

- Agave (*Agave americana*). One dose is 1/4–1 teaspoon/1–5 ml juice of the leaves.
- Alfalfa
- Amerikanerischer Schneeball (also available as Schneeball)
- Black cohosh (*Cimicifuga racemosa*)
- Black currant
- Black haw
- Bockshornklee
- Chaste tree (*Vitex agnus castus*)
- Cramp bark or guelder rose
- Dandelion
- Devil's club (*Chamalirium luteum*)
- Dong Quai/Dang Gui (*Angelica sinensis*)
- Fenugreek (*Trigonella foenumgraecum*) (good for hot flashes)
- Garden Sage (*Salvia officinalis*) (good for night sweats)
- Gemeines Kreuzkraut
- Ginseng (*Panax quinquefolium*)
- Groundsel
- Hopfen
- Hops
- Houblon grimpant (*Humulus lupulus*)
- Licorice (can be toxic in high doses, causing high blood pressure and water retention)
- Liferoot (*Senecio aureus*)
- Lowenzahn

- Luzerne
- Luzerne cultivee (*Medicago sativa*)
- Motherwort (*Leonurus cardiaca*) (good for night sweats)
- Nettle (*Urtica dioica* or *U. Urens*)
- Peony (frequently combines with Dong Quai/Dang Gui)
- Pomegranate (*Punica granatum*). (These seeds pack 1.7 grams of estrone for every 3 ounces. Just eat the seeds instead of spitting them out when you consume the fruit. Or make them into a smoothie in the blender. You can also rind them and infuse in oil to make your own estrogen cream.)
- Raspberry (Rubus species)
- Red clover (*Trifolium praetense*)
- Rose family (raspberry, strawberry, sweet briar, and hawthorn. Rosehips are an excellent source of flavonoids.)
- Sarsaparilla (*Smilax officinalis* or *S. regelii*) (Jamaican is considered best, with Mexican and Honduran following closely.)
- Saw palmetto (*Serenoa serrulata*)
- Schlangenwurzel
- Schwarze or Schwarze Johannisbeere
- Sweet briar or dog rose, hagrose, eglantier (*Rosa canina* or *R. pendulina*)
- Viorne obier (*Viburnum opulis*) or viburnum (*Viburnum prunifolium*)
- Wild yam (*Dioscorea villosa* and all 500 related species.) Progesterone cream derived from wild yam has been shown to reverse osteoporosis.
- Yarrow (*Achillea milefolium*)

herbal remedies

- Raspberry leaf. Best as an infusion (see Table 1.1). Nourishes the ovaries as well as the uterus, helps with erratic periods.
- Dong Quai/Dang Gui compound. As a tincture, this warms, regulates, and gently heals the entire reproductive system; especially useful if your irregular cycles are accompanied with premenstrual symptoms (PMS). (Note: Dong Quai can aggravate fibroids.)
- Liferoot Blossoms. As a tincture (see Table 1.2), 5 drops taken daily helps tonify the reproductive hormones, ovaries, uterus, adrenals, liver, and pituitary gland.
- Vitex. As a tincture, use one dropperful in a small glass of water 2 or 3 times daily for 6–8 weeks after every irregular period.

- Cinnamon bark (*Cinnamon zeylanicum*). This invigorates the blood, helps regulate the menstrual cycle, and helps with very heavy menstrual flows ("flooding"). As an infusion, sip a cup/250 ml of infusion, use 5–10 drops of tincture once or twice a day, gnaw on a cinnamon stick, or simply sprinkle cinnamon on everything.

for heavy menstrual flows

If you're coping with "flooding," or very heavy menstrual flows, it's important to consume roughly 2 mg iron from herbs or foods while the bleeding persists. This will help to prevent anemia. Iron is best in small doses throughout the day, rather than in one big gulp. Coffee, black tea, soy protein, egg yolks, bran, and calcium supplements over 250 mg can also impair iron absorption. Bleeding can be aggravated by aspirin, Midol, and larger doses of ascorbic acid (vitamin C supplements) because they thin the blood. In general, foods rich in bioflavonoids and carotene (brightly coloured fruits and veggies, for example) will help with blood loss.

herbal remedies

- Dandelion leaves. This is the best source of usable iron, containing roughly 30 grams of iron per ounce. Try them in a salad.
- Yellow dock root. An alcohol or vinegar tincture is best: 20 drops of alcohol tincture or 3 teaspoons/15 ml vinegar, taken in tea or water, gives you 1 mg iron to the blood.
- Lady's mantle (*Alchemilla vulgaris*). The alchemical weed controlled menstrual hemorrhage in virtually all of more than 300 women in a recent study.
- Wild yam root. As a tincture, 20–30 drops daily for the two weeks before your period can help reduce flow.

for hot flashes

Hot flashes deplete your body of vitamins B and C, magnesium and potassium. Red clover or oatstraw infusions will replace these lost nutrients. Vitamin B supplements (B2, B6, and B12), vitamin C, and vitamin E supplements are also helpful.

herbal remedies

It's suggested that you combine one of the following to help reduce the severity of hot flashes:

1. A "cooling" herb such as chickweed, elderflower, violet oatstraw, mint, seaweeds, all parts of the mallows (Malva species), and the flowers and leaves of any hibiscus.
2. A liver-nourishing herb, such as dandelion, yellow dock, Lowenzahn (*Taraxacum officinale*) root, Ho Shou Wu (*Polygonum multiflorum*) root (also sold as Fo-ti-tieng), or milk thistle (*Syllibum*); chicory (*Cichorium intybus*), and oatstraw.
3. A plant estrogen, such as black cohosh. (See above for a list of phytoestrogens.)

how to move

This section suggests activities, exercises, or specific movements to help reduce the severity of estrogen-loss discomforts. I've also selected some illustrations that outline postures which can help tone vaginal/pelvic muscles, including massaging specific acupressure points.

for hot flashes

exercise

Any kind of physical exercise can decrease hot flashes because it increases endorphin levels, which immediately counteract hot flashes. The recommended "dose" is 20 minutes three times a week.

1. Sit on the floor with knees bent. Partially extend your right leg, holding the middle of the sole of the foot with the index and middle fingers of your right hand. Hold, maintaining steady pressure for 1–3 minutes (see figure i).
2. Move your right hand to the point behind your ankle bone. Again, hold with steady pressure for 1–3 minutes and repeat both exercises on the left side (see figure ii).
3. With your left hand, hold the point on your right hand just outside of the fourth finger. Repeat on the left side.

For hot flashes, excessive menstrual bleeding, and other disturbances of the reproductive tract, try the following:

1. Lie on the floor with your knees bent. Place a knotted towel between your shoulder blades on the spine. Hold for 1–3 minutes.
2. With arms crossed across the chest, press your thumbs against the insides of your arms above the elbows. Hold for 1–3 minutes.
3. Move your left hand to the point at the base of your sternum or breastbone. Hold with steady pressure while you move your right hand to the point where your spine meets the back of your skull. Hold for 1–3 minutes.
4. Interlace your fingers and let them rest below your breasts. Press the tips of your fingers into your chest area with steady pressure. Hold for 1–3 minutes
5. Slide a knotted towel downward until it rests below your waistline. Apply steady pressure to the tailbone with your right hand, and to the tip of the pubic bone with your left hand. Hold for 1–3 minutes.
6. Lie on your back. Gently roll one, then the other shoulder inward, shortening the distance between your shoulder blades. Bring your knees to your chest, supporting your hips with your hands (see figure iii). Gently bring your legs up and over your body until they are resting on a chair behind you (see figure iv). Lift the spine by stretching the back muscles as much as possible. Breathe deeply and hold.
7. Lie on your back with your knees bent. Gently roll one, then the other shoulder inward, shortening the distance between your shoulder blades. With hands supporting your hips, slowly thrust your pelvis toward the ceiling. Breathe deeply, feeling the stretch all along the front of your body. Release.

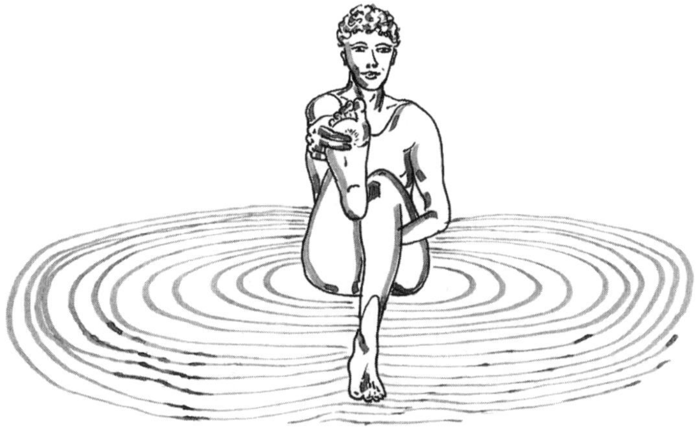

figure i

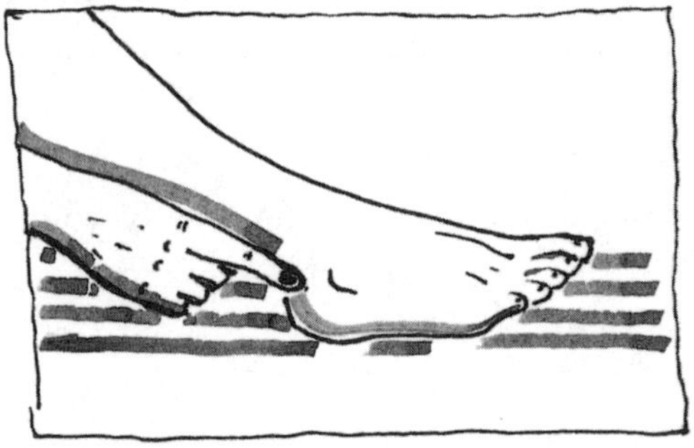

figure ii

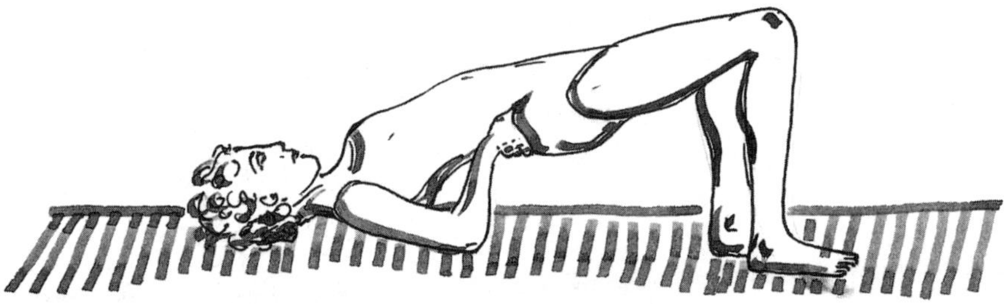

figure iii

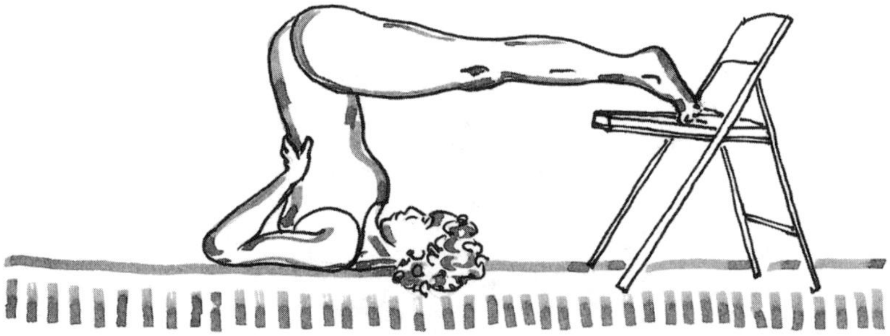

figure iv

aromatherapy

The following essential oils can help ease hot flashes. Use in a bath or diffuser:

- calamus/sweet flag
- basil
- thyme

other recommendations

- Use a hand-held fan.
- Use cologne, which is mostly alcohol and cooling.
- Bathe using 3 oz/80 ml rubbing alcohol.

for irregular menstrual periods

Both regular orgasms (through self- or partnered stimulation) and pelvic floor exercises can help maintain regular periods.

TABLE 1.1: HOW TO MAKE AN HERBAL INFUSION

A tea is a small amount of fresh or dried herb brewed for a short time. An infusion is a large amount of dried (not fresh) herb brewed for a long time. An infusion extracts more nutrients than a tincture and more medicinal qualities than a tea. Most infusions are short-lived; they're good for just two or three days.

Prepare infusions in pint/half-litre and quart/litre jars with tight lids. A teapot is not as good, but acceptable.

The usual dose of infusion is 1–2 cups a day, taken hot, chilled, or at room temperature. Infusions may be seasoned with sweeteners, tamari, milk, or any of the additions that please your taste. Infusions can be used as soup stocks, bath waters, hair rinses, facial washes, and so on.

SUMMARY OF INFUSION DATA

Roots/bark	1 oz./30 gm—pint/500 ml water	8 hours minimum
Leaves	1 oz/30 gm—quart/litre water	4 hours minimum
Flowers	1 oz/30 gm—quart/litre water	2 hours maximum
Seeds/berries	1 oz/30 gm—quart/litre water	30 minutes maximum

Source: Adapted from Susun S. Weed, *Wise Woman Ways: Menopausal Years.*

TABLE 1.2: HOW TO MAKE AN HERBAL TINCTURE

Fresh plant material steeped in alcohol makes alkaloid-rich (but nutrient-poor) remedies called tinctures. If you cannot find the fresh herb, you may use dried herb, but in my experience, only dried roots, seeds, and berries are worth the effort. Flowers and leaves lose too much in the drying. Tinctures remain effective for long periods of time and are easily transportable. Vinegar does not extract the same properties from plants as alcohol.

To tincture: identify and pick the plant. Chop the plant material coarsely; do not wash. Fill any size jar with the plant material, then pour 100-proof vodka or grain alcohol over it, filling the jar to the top. Cap tightly. Label with date and name of plant. Your tincture will be ready to use in six weeks but can stay there as long as you wish.

SUMMARY OF TINCTURE PROPORTIONS
*Tincture 1 oz/30 gm fresh plant in approximately 1 oz/30 ml spirit for six weeks
*Tincture 1 oz/30 gm dried plant material in 5 oz/150 ml spirit for six weeks

Source: Ibid.

***Note: Some of this text previously appeared in *The Gynecological Sourcebook*, 3rd Edition (1999, Lowell House), by same author.**

two

your heart of hearts

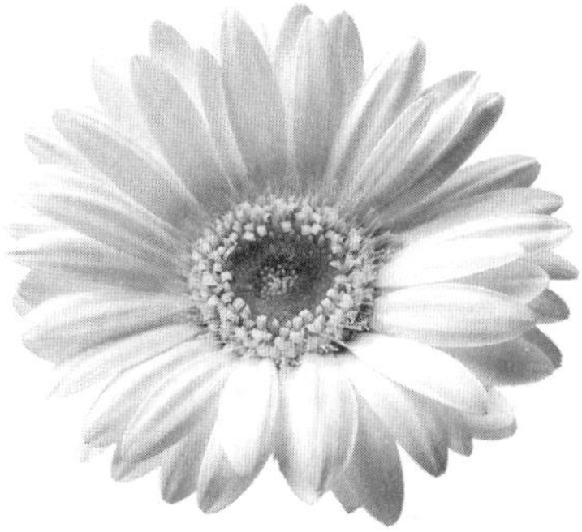

Heart disease is currently the number-one cause of death in postmenopausal women; in fact, more women die of heart disease than of lung cancer or breast cancer. Fifty per cent of all North Americans who die from heart attacks each year are women. But heart disease doesn't refer only to heart attacks; it refers to stroke, and a whole gamut of problems due to poor circulation, known in clinical circles as peripheral vascular disease (PVD) or, more plainly, blood circulation disease.

One of the reasons for such high death rates from heart attacks among women is medical ignorance: historically, most studies looking at heart disease excluded women, which led to a myth that more men than women die of heart disease. The truth is, more men die of heart attacks before age 50, while more women die of heart attacks after age 50, as a direct result of estrogen loss. Moreover, women who have had oophorectomies prior to natural menopause increase their risk of a heart attack by *eight times*. Since more women work outside the home than ever before, a number of experts cite stress as a huge contributing factor to increasing rates of heart disease in women.

Another problem is that women have different symptoms than men when it comes to heart disease, and so the "typical" warning signs we know about in men—angina, or chest pains—are often never present in women. In fact, chest pains in women are almost never related to heart disease. When symptoms of heart disease are not "male," many women are sent home to die, told that their heart attack is stress.

You're about to change all that. Never before have so many women been at risk for heart disease. As millions of women turn 50 in 2000, the medical community will be forced to recognize the unique warning signs of heart disease and heart attacks in women. This chapter outlines all the modifiable risk factors for heart disease and discusses the warning signs of a heart attack—in *women*. At the end of this chapter, What To Eat explains heart-smart diets and all of the heart-smart herbs available, while How To Move explains aerobic versus anaerobic activities, as well as postures that improve circulation and oxygen flow to the heart.

who's at risk for heart disease?

There are a number of *modifiable* risk factors that can predispose you to heart disease; that means risks that you can modify or alter, versus risks you can't change, such as age or family history.

smoking

Roughly half a million North Americans die of smoking-related illnesses each year. That's 20 per cent of *all* deaths from *all* causes. We already know that smoking causes lung cancer. But did you know that smokers are also twice as likely to develop heart disease? Include other factors, such as estrogen loss, and you're at enormous risk for heart disease if you're a postmenopausal smoker. A single cigarette affects your body within seconds, increasing heart rate, blood pressure, and the demand for oxygen. The greater the demand for oxygen (because of constricted blood vessels and carbon monoxide, a by-product of cigarettes) the greater the risk of heart disease.

Lesser-known long-term effects of smoking include a lowering of HDL, or "good" cholesterol, and damage to the lining of blood vessel walls, which paves the way for arterial plaque formation. In addition to increasing your risk for lung cancer and heart disease, smoking can lead to stroke, PVD, and a host of other cancers.

quitting smoking

The reason it's so hard to quit smoking is that it is difficult to deal with nicotine withdrawal symptoms. The symptoms of nicotine withdrawal begin within a few hours and peak at 24–48 hours after quitting. You may experience anxiety, irritability, hostility, restlessness, insomnia, and anger. However, take a look at some of the things you'll gain by quitting smoking: decreased risk of heart disease; decreased risk of cancer (that includes cancer of the lungs, esophagus, mouth, throat, pancreas, kidney, bladder, and cervix); lower heart rate and blood pressure; decreased risk of lung disease (bronchitis, emphysema); less constricted blood vessels; improved sense of smell and taste; whiter and prettier teeth; and fewer wrinkles.

Not everyone can quit cold turkey, although it's a strategy that many have used successfully. Some cold-turkey quitters report that keeping one package of cigarettes within reach lessons anxiety. Here are some other smoking-cessation methods:

Behavioural counselling: Behavioural counselling, either group or individual, can raise the rate of abstinence 20–25 per cent. This approach to smoking cessation aims to change the mental processes of smoking, reinforce the benefits of non-smoking, and teach skills to help the smoker avoid the urge to smoke.

Nicotine gum: Nicotine gum (for example Nicorette®) is now available over the counter in Canada and the United States. It helps you quit smoking by reducing nicotine cravings and withdrawal symptoms. Nicotine gum helps wean you from nicotine by allowing you to decrease the dosage gradually until you stop using it altogether, a process that usually takes about 12 weeks. The only disadvantage with this method is that it caters to the oral and addictive aspects of smoking, that is, rewarding the urge to smoke with a dose of nicotine.

Nicotine patch: Transdermal nicotine, or the "patch" (Habitrol®, Nicoderm®, Nicotrol®), doubles abstinence rates in former smokers. Most brands are now available over the counter in both Canada and the United States. With some products, a new patch is applied to a different area of dry, clean, hairless skin each morning and left on for the day. Other patches are designed to be worn a full 24 hours. However, the constant supply of nicotine to the bloodstream sometimes causes very vivid or disturbing dreams. You can also expect to feel a mild itching, burning, or tingling at the site of the patch when it is first applied. People are cautioned *not* to smoke while wearing the patch.

The nicotine patch works best when it is worn for at least 7–12 weeks, with a gradual decrease in strength (that is, nicotine). Many smokers find it effective because it allows them to tackle the psychological addiction to smoking before they are forced to deal with physical symptoms of withdrawal.

Nicotine inhaler: The nicotine inhaler (Nicotrol® Inhaler) delivers nicotine orally via inhalation from a plastic tube. Its success rate is about 28 per cent, similar to that of nicotine gum. It's available by prescription only in the U.S., and has yet to make its debut in Canada. Like nicotine gum, the inhaler mimics smoking behaviour by responding to each craving or urge to smoke, a feature which has both advantages and disadvantages to the smoker who wants to get over the physical symptoms of withdrawal. The nicotine inhaler should be used for a period of 12 weeks.

Nicotine nasal spray: Like nicotine gum and the nicotine patch, nicotine nasal spray reduces craving and withdrawal symptoms, allowing smokers to cut back gradually. One squirt delivers about 1 mg nicotine. In three clinical trials involving 730 patients, 31–35 per cent were not smoking at six months. This compares to an average of 12–15 per cent of smokers who were able to quit unaided.

The nasal spray has a couple of advantages over the gum and the patch: nicotine is rapidly absorbed across the nasal membranes, providing a kick that is more like the real thing; and the prompt onset of action, plus a flexible dosing schedule, benefits heavier smokers. Because the nicotine reaches the bloodstream so quickly, nasal sprays do have a greater potential for addiction than the slower-acting gum and patch. Nasal sprays are not yet available for use in Canada.

Bupropion: Bupropion (Zyban™) is appropriate for patients who have been unsuccessful using nicotine replacement therapy. Formerly prescribed as an antidepressant, Bupropion was discovered by accident: researchers knew that quitting smokers were often depressed, and so they began experimenting with the drug as a means to fight depression, not addiction.

Bupropion reduces the withdrawal symptoms associated with smoking cessation and can be used in conjunction with nicotine replacement therapy. Researchers suspect that Bupropion works directly in the brain to disrupt the addictive power of nicotine by affecting the same chemical neurotransmitters, or "messengers," such as dopamine, that nicotine does. The pleasurable aspect of addictive drugs like nicotine and cocaine is triggered by the release of dopamine. Smoking floods the brain with dopamine.

The *New England Journal of Medicine* published the results of a study of more than 600 smokers taking Bupropion. At the end of treatment, 44 per cent of those who took the highest dose of the drug (300 mg) were not smoking, compared to 19 per cent of the group who took a placebo. By the end of one year, 23 per cent of the 300 mg group and 12 per cent of the placebo group were still smoke-free. Using Zyban™ *with* nicotine replacement therapy seems to improve the quit rate a bit further. Four-week quit rates from the study were 23 per cent for placebo; 36 per cent for the patch; 49 per cent for Zyban™; and 58 per cent for the combination of Zyban™ and the patch.

Alternative therapies: Hypnosis, meditation, and acupuncture have helped some smokers quit. In the case of hypnosis and meditation, sessions may be private or part of a group smoking-cessation program.

obesity

If you weigh 20 per cent more than your ideal weight for your height and age, you are technically obese. It's not the weight that's the problem; it's the health conditions that usually accompany that weight, such as Type 2 diabetes (see chapter 7), high blood pressure, and high cholesterol, which can put you at risk for heart disease. For more about obesity, see chapter 3.

sedentary lifestyle

Women who are physically active have a 60–75 per cent lower risk of heart disease than inactive women. See How To Move for more details.

high cholesterol

Cholesterol is a whitish, waxy fat made in vast quantities by the liver. That's why liver or other organ meats are high in cholesterol. Cholesterol is needed to make hormones as well as cell membranes. If you have high cholesterol, the excess cholesterol in your blood can lead to narrowed arteries, which, in men, can definitely lead to a heart attack.

Saturated fat, discussed in detail in What To Eat, is often a culprit when it comes to high cholesterol. Sometimes, however, the highest levels of cholesterol are due to a genetic defect in the liver, which may not be modifiable.

The story of women and high cholesterol is still unfolding. You see, when it comes to high cholesterol, newer research shows that it is not as much of a risk factor for heart disease in women as it is for men. If you've already suffered a heart attack, following a low saturated-fat diet will help to lower "bad" cholesterol (LDL) and raise "good" cholesterol (HDL) levels. Similarly, if you smoke, have high blood pressure, are obese, have Type 2 diabetes (see chapter 7), or a family history of heart disease, following the low-fat, low-cholesterol diet will help improve your health, too.

In healthy women over age 65 with higher than normal cholesterol, who don't smoke and have no other risk factors for heart disease other than age, there's no clear benefit to lowering cholesterol or even worrying about it. We know, for example, that very few premenopausal women with high cholesterol ever develop heart disease, leading researchers to conclude that other factors are more significant for women than high cholesterol. So, while high cholesterol is *definitely* linked to male heart disease, it is *not* definitely linked to female heart disease, and in fact, may not even be a big deal. So most physicians will recommend a low-fat diet to women with other risk factors for heart disease because, in a nutshell, it can't hurt and will improve other health problems.

The current guidelines most physicians in North America follow when managing cholesterol in women are to encourage women over age 20 to begin a lower-cholesterol (meaning, low-saturated-fat diet—see What To Eat) if their cholesterol levels are 200 mg/dL or more. If you have very low "good" or "HDL" cholesterol levels (less than 35 mg/dL), your doctor should measure the "bad" or "LDL" cholesterol levels; an LDL level below 130 mg/dL is desirable. LDL levels of 130–159 mg/dL are borderline high. Levels of 160 mg/dL or above are high. Your doctor will probably recommend a low saturated-fat diet. If you already have heart disease, you should aim for LDL readings of about 100 mg/dL or less, which is lower than the guidelines for women without heart disease. In this case, your doctor may recommend that, in addition to a low saturated-fat diet, you also take a cholesterol-lowering drug, discussed below.

Cholesterol levels are checked through a simple blood test. You can also ask your pharmacist about the availability of home cholesterol tests.

If your blood cholesterol is between 200 and 239 mg/dL, so long as you don't smoke, are not obese, have normal blood pressure, are premenopausal, and do not have a family history of heart disease—you're fine! A high "total cholesterol" reading should always be followed up with an HDL–LDL analysis.

lowering cholesterol without drugs

By modifying your diet (see What To Eat) and exercising (see How To Move), you'll probably be able to lower your cholesterol without taking any medication.

Vitamin E has been shown to lower cholesterol, too, preventing the formation of arterial plaque. A 46 per cent drop in the incidence of heart attack was reported in a study of 87,000 nurses taking vitamin E. On the basis of that study, doctors now recommend a dosage of 100 IU (international units) daily.

As for vitamin C, we still don't know how much vitamin C is needed to reduce the risk of heart attack. Consumption of large amounts of vitamin C was associated with lower rates of coronary artery disease in an eight-year study at Brigham and Women's Hospital in Boston. Some experts recommend 10 mg vitamin C or more per day. (For more on heart-smart nutrients, see What To Eat.)

lowering cholesterol with drugs

For many, losing weight and modifying fat intake simply aren't enough to bring cholesterol levels down to optimal levels. You may be a candidate for one of the numerous cholesterol-lowering drugs that have hit the market in recent years. These medications, when combined with a low-fat, low-cholesterol diet, target the intestine, blocking food absorption and/or the liver, where they interfere with the processing of cholesterol. These are strong drugs, however, and ought to be a last resort after really giving a low-fat, low-cholesterol diet a chance. You might be given a combination of cholesterol-lowering medications to try with a low-cholesterol diet.

It's important to ask about all side effects accompanying your medication because they can include gastrointestinal problems, allergic reactions, blood disorders, and depression. One study found an unusually high rate of suicide and accidental trauma among male subjects taking cholesterol-lowering drugs. There have not been enough studies on women taking these drugs to truly know how these medications interact with women's health conditions. At any rate, here's what's available as of this writing. Please note only the generic drug names are listed.

Niacin. When taken properly, niacin is the best cholesterol treatment available. In 1986, the Coronary Drug Project, a National Institute of Health (NIH) study, found that prolonged use of niacin significantly reduced mortality rates among heart attack victims. It has since become one of the most popular cholesterol-lowering drugs on the market. Niacin, a water-soluble B vitamin, can lower LDL by 30 per cent, and triglyceride (blood fats) levels by as much as 55 per cent. It also increases HDL by about 35 per cent. Also known as nicotinic acid, niacin must be taken in large doses (1–3 mg/day) in order to be effective. Because the dosage is up to 76 times higher than the recommended daily allowance, side effects are common. Many patients experience itching, flushing, and panic attacks. Switching to slow-release capsules, taking an aspirin 30 minutes before ingesting the medication, or taking it on a full stomach might help alleviate some of these symptoms. Niacin can aggravate both stomach ulcers and diabetes.

Statins. Statins like Mevacor® and Zocar hinder the liver's ability to produce cholesterol, keeping LDL levels to a minimum while increasing levels of HDL. When combined with the proper diet, statins can reduce your risk of death from heart disease by as much as 40 per cent. However, certain lovastatins (Zocar) have been known to cause liver damage, muscle pain, and weakness.

Cholestyramine. Cholestyramine helps the body eliminate cholesterol through the gut. It is considered the safest cholesterol-lowering drug; it has also been around the longest. A National Institute of Health study in the early 1980s demonstrated that cholestyramine decreases heart attack deaths by lowering cholesterol levels. In fact, for each 1 per cent drop in the cholesterol levels of participants, there was a 2 per cent drop in death rates. Pretty impressive when you consider that the average decline in blood cholesterol was 25 per cent. Although cholestyramine reduces LDL cholesterol, it can sometimes raise triglyceride levels. It can also trigger a host of side effects, the most unpleasant of which is *really bad* gas. Cholestyramine interferes with the effectiveness of digitalis, diuretics, the blood thinner Warfarin, fat-soluble vitamins, and beta-blockers. It can also lead to gallstones. Cholestyramine should be taken in the morning and at bedtime.

Gemfibrozil. Gemfibrozil lowers cholesterol and triglyceride levels in the blood. The rate of coronary artery disease among 4,000 men with high cholesterol involved in a Finnish study dropped 34 per cent when they were put on gemfibrozil. Gemfibrozil should be taken in 600 mg tablets twice daily.

Probucol. Probucol can cut LDL levels by as much as 15 per cent, but it also lowers HDL levels. Lately, Probucol is generating new interest among doctors because it is also a powerful cancer-fighting antioxidant. LDL creates arterial plaque through a change in its molecular make-up. This change is called oxidation, and an antioxidant like Probucol can help to prevent oxidation from happening.

Arginine. Studies suggest that this amino acid lowers cholesterol levels and improves coronary blood flow by acting as an antioxidant and maintaining elasticity in blood vessel tissues. Arginine is currently available without a prescription.

Coenzyme Q_{10}. Japanese and European practitioners love this powerful antioxidant, but more studies are needed to prove its reputed effect on arterial plaque.

high blood pressure

About 12 per cent of all North American adults suffer from hypertension, or high blood pressure. What, exactly, is blood pressure? The blood flows from the heart into the arteries (blood vessels), pressing against the artery walls. The simplest way to explain this is to think about a liquid-soap dispenser. When you want soap, you need to pump it out by pressing down on the little dispenser pump, the "heart" of the dispenser. The liquid soap is the "blood" and the little tube through which the soap flows is the "artery." The pressure that's exerted on the wall of the tube is therefore the "blood pressure."

When the tube is hollow and clean, you needn't pump very hard to get the soap; it comes out easily. But when the tubing in your dispenser gets narrower as a result of old, hardened, gunky liquid soap blocking it, you have to pump down much harder to get any soap, while the force the soap exerts against the tube is increased. Obviously, this is a simplistic explanation of a very complex problem, but essentially the narrowing of the arteries, created by higher blood pressure, forces your heart to work harder to pump the blood. If this goes on too long, your heart muscle enlarges and becomes weaker, which can lead to a heart attack. Higher pressure can also weaken the walls of your blood vessels, which can cause a stroke.

The term hyper*tension* refers to the tension or force exerted on your artery walls. ("Hyper" means "too much," as in "too much tension.") Blood pressure is measured in two readings: X over Y. The X is the *systolic pressure*, which is the pressure that occurs during the heart's contraction. The Y is the *diastolic pressure*, which is the pressure that occurs when the heart rests between contractions. In "liquid soap" terms, the systolic pressure occurs when you press the pump down; the diastolic pressure occurs when you release your hand from the pump and allow it to rise back to its "resting" position.

Normal blood pressure readings are 120 over 80 (120/80). Readings of 140/90 or higher are generally considered borderline, although for some people this is still considered a normal reading. For the general population, 140/90 is "lecture time," when your doctor will begin to counsel you about dietary and lifestyle habits. By 160/100, many people are prescribed a hypertensive drug, which is designed to lower blood pressure.

know the causes of high blood pressure

The most common causes of high blood pressure are obesity, inactivity, and stress.

High blood pressure is also exacerbated by tobacco and alcohol consumption, and too much sodium or salt in the diet. (People of African descent tend to be more salt-sensitive.)

If high blood pressure runs in the family, you're considered at greater risk of developing hypertension. High blood pressure can also be caused by kidney disorders or pregnancy, known as pregnancy-induced hypertension. Medications are also common culprits. Estrogen-containing medications (such as oral contraceptives), non-steroidal anti-inflammatory drugs (NSAIDs), such as ibuprofen, nasal decongestants, cold remedies, appetite suppressants, certain antidepressants and other drugs can all increase blood pressure. Be sure to check with your pharmacist.

lowering your blood pressure without drugs

There are a number of ways you can lower your blood pressure without taking medication. Try some of the following lifestyle changes: change your diet and begin exercising (see What To Eat and How To Move); limit your alcohol consumption to no more than 2 oz of liquor or 8 oz of wine or 24 oz of beer per day, and lower still, for liver health; limit your salt intake to about 1–1/2 teaspoons per day. Cut out all foods high in sodium, such as canned soups, pickles, soy sauce, and so on. Some canned soups contain 1,000 mg of sodium, for example. That's a lot!; increase your intake of calcium or dairy products and potassium (for example, bananas). Some still-unproven studies suggest that people with hypertension are calcium- and potassium-deficient; and lower your stress levels. Studies show that by lowering stress, your blood pressure decreases.

lowering your blood pressure with drugs

If you can't lower your blood pressure through lifestyle changes, you may be a candidate for some of the following blood pressure-lowering drugs:

Diuretics. Diuretics are the most commonly used blood pressure medication. Also known as water pills, diuretics work by flushing excess water and salt (often 2–4 pounds' worth!) out of your system. However, diuretics may actually increase the risk of heart attack by leaching potassium salts needed by the heart; and the heart may respond to blocked nerve signals by trying harder and harder, until it fails. Another common side effect of diuretic therapy is low potassium. Levels of potassium tend to drop when diuretics replace the low-fat diet you've worked so hard to maintain. If you make sure not to substitute one therapy for another, diuretics will not affect your potassium levels. Other possible side effects include increased blood sugar and cholesterol levels.

Beta-blockers. Beta-blockers alter the way hormones like adrenaline control blood pressure. They slow the heart rate by decreasing the strength of the heart's contractions. Beta-blockers are most often used by young people and people with coronary artery disease. Possible side effects include fatigue and an increase in blood sugar and cholesterol levels.

Centrally acting agents. These drugs act through centres in the brain to slow the heart rate and relax the blood vessels. Possible side effects include stuffy nose, dry mouth, and drowsiness.

Vasodilators. Vasodilators dilate, or relax, the blood vessels, thereby reducing blood pressure.

Ace-inhibitors. Ace-inhibitors lower blood pressure by preventing the formation of a hormone called angiotensin II, which causes the blood vessels to narrow. Ace-inhibitors are also used to treat heart failure. Possible side effects include cough and swelling of the face and tongue.

Alpha-blocking agents. Alpha-blocking agents block the effects of adrenaline, allowing the blood vessels to relax. Blood pressure decreases with treatment, as does cholesterol. You may also notice an increase in HDL cholesterol. A possible side effect is blood pressure variation when standing as opposed to reclining.

Calcium-channel blockers. Calcium-channel blockers limit the amount of calcium entering the cells, allowing the blood vessels to relax. Possible side effects include ankle swelling, flushing, constipation, and indigestion.

type 2 diabetes

If you have Type 2 diabetes, your risk of a heart attack or stroke is at least four times greater than in the general population. In fact, Type 2 diabetes is referred to as "a heart attack about to happen." See chapter 7 for more information about controlling this disease if you've been diagnosed. Preventing Type 2 diabetes can be done by following the heart-smart diet and exercise program outlined at the end of this chapter in What To Eat and How To Move.

the role of stress

Heart disease is also believed to be triggered by stress. Before you can look at what you can do to manage your stress, the first order of business is understanding what, exactly, stress is.

Generally, stress is defined as a negative emotional experience associated with biological changes that allow you to adapt to it. In response to stress, your adrenal glands pump out stress hormones that speed up your body: your heart rate increases, your blood sugar levels increase so that glucose can be diverted to your muscles in case you have to "run." This is known as the "fight or flight" response

The problem with stress hormones in the 21st century is that the fight or flight response isn't usually necessary since most of our stress is emotional. Occasionally, we may want to flee from a bank robbery or mugger, but most of us just want to flee from our jobs or our kids! In other words, our stress hormones actually put a physical strain on our bodies, and can lower our resistance to disease, which can impact the body from head to toe. As a result, we can suffer from stress-related headaches, gastrointestinal problems, bladder problems, heart problems, back pain, high blood pressure, and high cholesterol.

good stress

Good things come from good stress, even though it feels stressful or bad in the short term. Stress challenges us to stretch ourselves beyond our capabilities, which is what makes us meet deadlines, push the envelope, and invent creative solutions to our problems. Examples of good stress include challenging projects; positive life-changing events (moving, changing jobs, or ending unhealthy relationships); confronting fears, illness, or people who make us feel bad (this is one of those bad-in-the-short-term/good-in-the-long-term situations).

Essentially, whenever a stressful event triggers emotional, intellectual, or spiritual growth, it is a good stress. It is often not the event as much as your response to the event that determines whether it is a "good" or "bad" stress. For example, the death of a loved one can sometimes lead to personal growth because we may see something about ourselves we did not see before—new resilience, for example. So even a death can be a good stress, though we grieve and are sad in the short term.

bad stress

When no growth occurs from a stressful event, it is "bad stress." Bad stress results from boredom and stagnation. When negative events don't seem to yield anything positive in the long term, but more of the same, the stress can lead to chronic and debilitating health problems. This is not to say that we can't get sick from good stress, too, but when there is nothing positive from the stress, it has a much more negative effect on our health. Examples of bad stress include stagnant jobs or relationships, disability from terrible accidents or diseases, or long-term unemployment. These kind of situations can lead to depression, low self-esteem, and a host of physical illnesses.

managing stress

What we *perceive* as stressful has great bearing on how well we manage it. Women who are already overloaded will feel more stress as well. In general, we feel stress when we experience negative events; uncontrollable or unpredictable events; or ambiguous events, versus clear-cut situations.

Moreover, how stressed you become has much to do with your personality. For example, if you have a negative outlook on life, you'll probably feel more stress than someone who enjoys a positive outlook. Some women like to find meaning in uncontrollable events, which gives them a sense of control; others like the challenge of difficult situations.

Our strategies for coping also vary. Some women like to avoid the stress and minimize the problem. This has short-term benefits but, in the long term, the stress does not disappear. Women who confront the stress in the short term will feel more anxious at first, but will probably feel relief in the long term when the stress is dealt with. People who suffer less stress-related health problems use humour, spiritual support, and social support to deal with stress.

If the following statements sound like you, you're probably not managing stress very well.

1. I tend to imagine all of the terrible things that could possibly happen to me rather than just concerning myself with the stressful situation at hand.
2. I stop what I'm doing and devote all my energy toward fixing the problem immediately. (I might as well do this because, if I don't, I will just drive myself crazy with worry).
3. I relive my latest crisis in my mind over and over again...even after it's been solved.
4. I actually picture the stressful situation in my mind's eye, as well as picturing the worst possible outcome.
5. I get the feeling that I'm losing control over everything.
6. I feel a sinking feeling in my stomach, my mouth getting dry, my heart pounding, or my neck and shoulder muscles tightening.
7. I have trouble falling asleep at night and wake up in the middle of the night.
8. I tend to make mountains out of molehills. (I sort of know I'm doing this, but I can't stop myself.)
9. I have difficulty speaking, or notice my hands and/or fingers trembling.
10. I notice my thoughts racing.

stress reduction

Since so many of the health problems discussed in this chapter are manifestations of stress, what can you do to lower your stress—*realistically*? Being told to simply "take things easy and relax" is not a solution, because indeed, if we weren't so stressed, we *would* relax!

Stress reduction depends entirely on the source of your stress. The only way to control stress that appears to be beyond your control is to shift your response to stress. And for many women, this takes time, and may require some work with a qualified counsellor.

If you are the source of your own stress because you're too hard on yourself, or are a perfectionist, you need to work on lowering your self-expectations and forgiving yourself for not being perfect. Again, working with a therapist or counsellor may help. In the meantime, consider the following suggestions for reducing some sources of daily stress:

1. Isolate the exact source of stress and see if there's a solution. Taking the time to think about what, in fact, the real problem is can work wonders.
2. See the humour in difficult situations, and try to look at lessons learned instead of beating yourself up.
3. When times get tough, surround yourself with supportive people: close friends and family members.
4. Don't take things so personally. When people don't respond to you the way you'd like, consider other factors. For instance, maybe the other person has problems unrelated to you that are affecting his/her behaviour.
5. Focus on something pleasant in the future, such as a vacation, and allow yourself time to daydream and plan.
6. Just say no. If you can't take on that "small favour" or extra task, just politely say, "I'd love to, but it's impossible..."
7. Take time out for yourself. Spend some time alone and block everyone out once a week or so. This is a great time to go for a long walk and get in a little exercise.
8. Make some lists. Some people find listmaking really helps; others find it is just another chore. But if you haven't been a listmaker, try it. It might help you get a little more focused and organized on the tasks at hand.
9. Investigate some alternative healing systems, such as massage, Chinese exercises such as qi gong (pronounced "chi kong") or Tai Chi.
10. Eat a balanced diet.

signs of a woman's heart attack

For women, the symptoms of heart disease, and even an actual heart attack, can be vague, seemingly unrelated to heart problems. Signs of heart disease in women include some surprising symptoms, some of which may be masked by thyroid problems. On the other hand, a woman experiencing some of these symptoms may be worried she is having a heart attack when, in fact, her symptoms are purely thyroid-related. So please review the following list of signs carefully:

- Shortness of breath and/or fatigue
- Jaw pain (often masked by arthritis and joint pain)
- Pain in the back of the neck (often masked by arthritis or joint pain)

- Pain down the right or left arm
- Back pain (often masked by arthritis and joint pain)
- Sweating (ladies—have your thyroid checked; this is a classic sign of an overactive thyroid gland; if you're diabetic, test your blood sugar—you may be low)
- Fainting
- Palpitations (ladies—again, have your thyroid checked; this is also a classic symptom of an overactive thyroid)
- Bloating (after menopause, would you believe this is a sign of coronary artery blockage?)
- Heartburn, belching, or other gastrointestinal pain (this is often a sign of an actual heart attack in women)
- Chest "heaviness" between the breasts (this is how women experience chest pain; some describe it as a "sinking feeling" or burning sensation). Also described as an "aching, throbbing, or a squeezing sensation"; "hot poker tab between the chest" or feeling like your heart jumps into your throat
- Sudden swings in blood sugar
- Vomiting
- Confusion

Clearly, there are lots of other causes for the symptoms on this list. But it's important that your doctor includes heart disease as a possible cause, rather than dismissing it because your symptoms are not "male" (which your doctor may refer to as "typical").

Diagnostic tests that can confirm heart disease in women include a manual exam, in which the doctor examines you with a stethoscope; an electrocardiogram; an exercise stress test; an echocardiogram; as well as a myriad of imaging tests that may use radioactive substances to take pictures of the heart.

preventing or reversing heart disease

If you're diagnosed with heart disease, the "cure" is prevention or reversal through diet (see What To Eat), exercise (see How To Move), and protection through HRT, cholesterol-lowering drugs and possibly blood pressure-lowering drugs. In fact, it's estimated that roughly 90 per cent of all heart disease is preventable with lifestyle changes.

HRT and heart disease

Heart attack statistics are much lower in premenopausal women than in postmenopausal women. In the premenopause age group, men outperform women by a vast degree. However, 10 to 15 years after menopause, women equal men in terms of heart attacks. To date, most research shows that estrogen will *protect* women from heart disease.

It's also important to review these studies in the proper context. First, the women who are selected for this research are generally upper-middle-class and educated: two major factors that appear to decrease the risk of heart disease anyway. Second, women who take estrogen are usually healthier, and are more willing to make other lifestyle changes that will lower their risk, such as improving their diet or quitting smoking.

Finally, some animal research revealed that the progesterone added to HRT may have the opposite influence on HDL as estrogen. If you decide to go on HRT for strictly the heart benefit, it is a good idea to have your cholesterol level checked before you start the therapy, as a baseline, and then get your levels checked after you're on HRT for about three months. If there's no improvement in your cholesterol levels, you might want to review your decision with your doctor.

However, the heart benefits seen with estrogen is only true if the estrogen is taken orally, not in a patch or vaginal cream. In order for the estrogen to work its magic with HDL, it needs to be metabolized in the liver.

Finally, estrogen will not counteract a poor diet and lifestyle. If you smoke, drink excessively, are under tremendous stress, eat copious amounts of the wrong foods (see chapter 3), or come from a heart attack family, don't expect estrogen alone to shield you from heart disease.

lifestyle changes

Use the information in the following two sections to make the necessary lifestyle changes for heart health. Quitting smoking and making an attempt to reduce stress will also prevent cardiovascular diseases.

what to eat

The way to a woman's heart is through her stomach, too. The most dramatic prevention of heart disease starts with a heart-smart, low-fat diet. Often what we think is low-fat is deceiving, especially when it comes to trying to decipher complex nutrition labels. This section tells you everything you need to know about fat (and wish you didn't!).

understanding fat

Fat is technically known as *fatty acids*, which are crucial nutrients for our cells. We cannot live without fatty acids, or fat. If you looked at each fat molecule carefully, you'd find three different kinds of fatty acids on it: saturated (solid), monounsaturated (less solid, with the exception of olive and peanut oils), and polyunsaturated (liquid) fatty acids. The term "unsaturated fat" refers to either monounsaturated or polyunsaturated fats.

These three fatty acids combine with glycerol to make what's chemically known as triglycerides. Each fat molecule is a link chain made up of glycerol, carbon atoms and hydrogen atoms. The more hydrogen atoms that are on that chain, the more saturated or solid the fat. The liver breaks down fat molecules by secreting bile (stored in the gallbladder)—its sole function. The liver also makes cholesterol. Too much saturated fat may cause your liver to overproduce cholesterol, while the triglycerides in your bloodstream will rise, perpetuating the problem.

Fat is therefore a good thing—in moderation. But like all good things, most of us want too much of it. Excess dietary fat is by far the most damaging element in the Western diet. A gram of fat contains twice the calories as the same amount of protein or carbohydrate. Decreasing the fat in your diet and replacing it with more grain products, vegetables, and fruit is the best way to lower your risk of colon cancer and cardiovascular diseases.

Fat in the diet comes from meats, dairy products, and vegetable oils. Other sources of fat include coconuts (60 per cent fat), peanuts (78 per cent fat), and avocados (82 per cent fat). There are different kinds of fatty acids in these sources of fats: saturated, monounsaturated, and polyunsaturated (which, again, is what is meant by the term "unsaturated fat"). And then there is a fourth kind of fat in our diets: trans-fatty acids. This is a factory-made fat that is found in margarines, for example. (See pages 53–55 for details.)

To cut through all this big fat jargon, you can boil down fat into two categories: "harmful fats" and "helpful fats," which the media often defines as "good fats/bad fats."

harmful fats

The following are harmful fats because they can increase your risk of cardiovascular problems, as well as many cancers, including colon and breast cancers. These are fats that are fine in moderation but harmful in excess (and harmless if not eaten at all):

- *Saturated fats.* These fats are solid at room temperature and stimulate cholesterol production in your body. In fact, the way that saturated fat looks prior to ingesting it is the way it will look when it lines your arteries. Foods high in saturated fat include: processed meat, fatty meat, lard, butter, margarine, solid vegetable shortening, chocolate and tropical oils (coconut oil is more than 90 per cent saturated). Saturated fat should be consumed only in very low amounts.
- *Trans-fatty acids.* These are factory-made fats that behave just like saturated fat in your body. (See below.)

helpful fats

The following are helpful fats because the can actually protect against certain health problems, including heart disease. These are fats that you are encouraged to use more frequently in your diet. In fact, nutritionists suggest that you substitute harmful fats with these:

- *Unsaturated fat.* This fat is partially solid or liquid at room temperature. The more liquid the fat, the more polyunsaturated it is, which, in fact, *lowers* your cholesterol levels. This group of fats comprise monounsaturated fats and polyunsaturated fats. Sources of unsaturated fats include vegetable oils (canola, safflower, sunflower, corn) and seeds and nuts. Unsaturated fats come from plants, with the exception of tropical oils, such as coconut. (See above.)
- *Fish fats (a.k.a. omega-3 fatty acids).* The fats naturally present in fish that swim in cold waters, known as omega-3 fatty acids or fish oils, are all polyunsaturated. Again, polyunsaturated fats are good for you: they lower cholesterol levels, are crucial for brain tissue, and protect against heart disease. Look for cold-water fish like mackerel, albacore tuna, salmon, and sardines.

factory-made fats—trans-fatty acids

An assortment of factory-made fats have been introduced into our diet, courtesy of food producers who are trying to give us the taste of fat without all the calories of saturated fats. Unfortunately, factory-made fats offer their own bag of horrors. That's because when a fat is made in a factory, it becomes a trans-fatty acid, a harmful fat that not only raises the level of "bad" cholesterol (LDL) in your bloodstream, but also lowers the amount of "good" cholesterol (HDL) that's already there.

How, exactly, does a trans-fatty acid come into being? Trans-fatty acids are what you get when you make a liquid oil, such as corn oil, into a more solid or spreadable substance, such as margarine. Trans-fatty acids, you might say, are the "road to hell, paved with good intentions." Someone, way back when, thought that if you could take the "good fat"—unsaturated fat—and solidify it so it could double as butter or lard, you could eat the same things without missing the spreadable fat. That sounds like a great idea. Unfortunately, to make an unsaturated liquid fat more solid, you have to add *hydrogen* to its molecules. The process that converts liquid fat to semi-solid fat is known as hydrogenation. That ever-popular chocolate bar ingredient "hydrogenated palm oil" is a classic example of a trans-fatty acid. Hydrogenation also prolongs the shelf life of a fat, such as polyunsaturated fats, which can oxidize when exposed to air, causing rancid odors or flavours. Deep-frying oils used in the restaurant trade are generally hydrogenated.

what's wrong with trans-fatty acid?

Trans-fatty acid is sold as a polyunsaturated or monounsaturated fat with a line of advertising copy such as: "Made from polyunsaturated vegetable oil." Except in your body, it is treated as a *saturated* fat. So, really, trans-fatty acids are a saturated fat in disguise. The advertiser may, in fact, say that the product contains "no saturated fat" or is "healthier" than the comparable animal or tropical oil product with saturated fat. So be careful out there: read your labels. The magic word you're looking for is "hydrogenated." If the product label lists a variety of unsaturated fats (monounsaturated X oil, polyunsaturated Y oil, and so on), keep reading. If the word "hydrogenated" appears, count that product as a saturated fat; your body will!

margarine versus butter

There's an old tongue twister: "Betty Botter bought some butter that made the batter bitter; so Betty Botter bought more butter that made the batter better." Are we making our batters bitter or better with margarine? It depends.

Since the news of trans-fatty acids broke in the late 1980s, margarine manufacturers began to offer some less "bitter" margarines; some contain no hydrogenated oils, while others contain much smaller amounts. Margarines with less than 60–80 per cent oil (9–11 grams of fat) will contain 1.0–3.0 grams of trans-fatty acids per serving, compared to butter, which is 53 per cent saturated fat. You might say it's a choice between a bad fat and a *worse* fat.

It's also possible for a liquid vegetable oil to retain a high concentration of unsaturated fat when it's been partially hydrogenated. In this case, your body will metabolize this as some saturated fat and some unsaturated fat.

cutting down on carbs

Fat is not the only thing that can make you fat: *what about carbohydrates?* You see, a diet high in carbohydrates can also make you fat. That's because carbohydrates—meaning starchy stuff, such as rice, pasta, breads, or potatoes—can be stored as fat when eaten in excess.

Carbohydrates can be simple or complex. Simple carbohydrates are found in any food that has natural sugar (honey, fruits, juices, vegetables, milk) and anything that contains table sugar.

Complex carbohydrates are more sophisticated foods that are made up of larger molecules, such as grain foods, starches, and foods high in fibre.

Normally, all carbs convert into glucose when you eat them. Glucose is the technical term for "simplest sugar." All your energy comes from glucose in your blood—also known as blood glucose or blood sugar—your body fuel. When your blood sugar is used up, you feel weak and tired...and hungry. But what happens when you eat more carbohydrates than your body can use? Your body will store those extra carbs as fat. What we also know is that the rate at which glucose is absorbed by your body from carbohydrates is affected by other parts of your meal, such as the protein, fibre, and fat. If you're eating only carbohydrates and no protein or fat, for example, they will convert into glucose more quickly, to the point where you may feel mood swings, as your blood sugar rises and dips.

Nutrition experts advise that you should consume roughly 50–55 per cent carbohydrates; 15–20 per cent protein, and less than 30 per cent fat daily for a healthy diet.

cutting down on factory-added sugars

What you have to watch out for is added sugar; these are sugars that manufacturers add to foods during processing or packaging. Foods containing fruit juice concentrates, invert sugar, regular corn syrup, honey or molasses, hydrolyzed lactose syrup or high-fructose corn syrup (made out of highly concentrated fructose through the hydrolysis of starch), all have added sugars. Many people don't realize, however, that pure, *unsweetened* fruit juice is still a potent source of sugar, even when it contains no added sugar. Extra lactose (naturally occurring sugar in milk products), dextrose (edible glucose), and maltose (naturally occurring sugar in grains) are also contained in many foods. In other words, the products may have naturally occurring sugars anyway, and then *more* sugar is thrown in to enhance consistency, taste, and so on. The best way to know how much sugar is in a product is to look at the nutritional label for "carbohydrates."

understanding fibre

Fibre is the part of a plant your body can't digest, which comes in the form of both water soluble fibre (which dissolves in water) and water insoluble fibre (which does not dissolve in water but instead absorbs water); this is what's meant by "soluble" and "insoluble" fibre.

Soluble and insoluble fibre do differ, but they are equally good things. Soluble fibre, somehow, lowers the "bad" cholesterol in your body. Experts aren't entirely sure how soluble fibre works its magic, but one popular theory is that it gets mixed into the bile the liver secretes, and forms a type of gel that traps the building blocks of cholesterol, thus lowering LDL levels. It's akin to a spiderweb trapping smaller insects.

Sources of soluble fibre include oats or oat bran, legumes (dried beans and peas), some seeds, carrots, oranges, bananas, and other fruits. Soybeans are also high sources of soluble fibre. Studies show that people with very high cholesterol have the most to gain by eating soybeans. Soybean is also a phytoestrogen (see page 24) that is believed to lower the risks of estrogen-related cancers, as well as lower the incidence of estrogen-loss symptoms associated with menopause (see chapter 1).

Insoluble fibre doesn't affect your cholesterol levels at all, but it regulates your bowel movements. (See chapter 5.) Whole-grain breads are good sources of insoluble fibre (flax bread is particularly good because flaxseeds are a source of soluble fibre, too). The problem is understanding what is truly "whole grain." For example, there is an assumption that because bread is dark or brown, it's more nutritious; this isn't so. In fact, many brown breads are simply enriched white breads dyed with molasses. (The term "enriched" on the food label means that nutrients lost during processing have been replaced.) High-fibre pita breads and bagels are available, but you have to search for them. A good rule is to simply look for the phrase "whole wheat," which means that the wheat is, indeed, whole.

alcohol

Alcohol delivers about 7 calories per gram or 150 calories per drink. It's the sugar *in* that alcoholic beverage that can also pack in more calories. That said, alcohol has been proven to raise your "good" cholesterol (HDL). This fact was discovered in the late 1980s when researchers probed why France, with all its rich food, had such low rates of heart disease. It was the wine; red wine, in particular, was shown to decrease the risk of cardiovascular disease. But any alcohol will do this. So it's okay to have this stuff, so long as you drink it in moderation.

herbs for the heart

Herbs that are good for the uterus are also good for the heart. Plants that strengthen the uterus and the heart are either green or red, such as hawthorn, rose, strawberry, raspberry, and motherwort. As a rule, if you're experiencing hot flashes or night sweats, these herbs can trigger heart palpitations. Drinking lots of water, mineral-rich herbal infusions, fresh grape juice or grapes will help you retain fluids and reduce palpitations.

to nourish and tone the heart

- Wheat germ oil. One or more tablespoons/15ml daily.
- Vitamin E oil. One or more tablespoons daily.
- Flaxseed (*Linum usitatissimum*). Also known as linseed, flaxseed is considered the best heart oil, but only if it is absolutely fresh and taken uncooked; 1–3 teaspoons/5–15 ml of flaxseed oil first thing in the morning is recommended. You can also grind the seeds and sprinkle them on cereals or salads. You can also soak flaxseeds in water and drink the whole thing first thing in the morning.
- Fresh pressed oils of borage seed or black currant seed.
- Plantain, lamb's quarter, or amaranth.
- Hawthorn berry. As a tincture, 25–40 drops of the berry tincture up to 4 times a day. Expect results no sooner than 6–8 weeks.
- Seaweed.
- Carotene-rich foods. Look for bright-coloured fruits and vegetables. The richer the colour, the richer they are in carotene.
- Garlic (*Allium sativum*). Greatest heart benefits come from eating it raw, but you can also purchase deodorized caplets.

- Lemon balm. Steep a handful of fresh leaves in a glass of white wine for an hour or so and drink it with dinner. Or make lemon balm vinegar to use on salads.
- Dandelion root. As a tincture, 10–15 drops with meals.
- Ginseng (*Panax quinquefolium*). Chew on the root or use 5–40 drops of tincture.
- Motherwort (*Leonurus cardiaca*). Use a tincture of the flowering tops, 5–15 drops several times a day as needed.

To calm the heart

- Rose flower essence.
- Hawthorn (*Crataegus*). Try 25–40 drops up to four times a day. Slow-acting, it requires about a month of use before you see results.
- Motherwort. As a tincture, 10–20 drops with meals and before bed, or 25–50 drops for immediate relief of palpitations.
- Valerian root. As a tea or tincture.
- Ginger root tea, hot or cold. (Note: May aggravate hot flashes and heavy menstrual flows.)
- A piece of real licorice root to slow palpitations.

blood-thinning herbs

Blood thinners, such as aspirin, can reduce the incidence of stroke or heart attack. A daily spoonful of vinegar made from the leaves, buds, and/or flowers of any of the following herbs can give you the same health benefits of aspirin, but also help calcium absorption and improve digestion: alfalfa; birch; sweet clover; bedstraws; poplar; red clover; willow; wintergreen; black haw. (Note: Do not take blood-thinning herbs if you are bleeding heavily, or require surgery.)

supplements

- Niacin. Recommended dose is 500 mg with meals (three times a day). This can initially cause a hot flash-like flush for about 30 minutes after you ingest it. The more regularly you take niacin, the less often you will flush, if at all. Discontinue use if you feel nauseated or experience gastrointestinal distress.
- Magnesium. To slow palpitations. Check with your doctor about appropriate dosages.

herbs to lower blood pressure

- Hawthorn. As a tincture, 10–20 drops 3 times daily
- Motherwort. As a tincture, 10–20 drops 3 times daily.
- Dandelion root. As a tincture, 10–15 drops with meals.
- Potassium. 80–85 per cent of people who eat six portions of potassium-rich foods daily will reduce their need for blood pressure–lowering medication by half or more.
- Raw garlic. Just 1/2 to 1 clove of raw garlic a day can dramatically reduce your blood pressure. Mince it raw into a variety of dishes, including eggs, rice, or potatoes.
- Ginseng. Any amount.
- Seaweed. Any amount.

how to move

If you look up the word "aerobic" in the dictionary, what you'll find is the chemistry definition: "living in free oxygen." This is certainly correct; we are all aerobes—beings that require oxygen to live. Some bacteria, for example, are *anaerobic*; they can exist in an environment without oxygen. All that jumping around and fast movement is done to create faster breathing, so we can take more oxygen into our bodies.

Why are we doing this? Because the blood contains *oxygen*! The faster your blood flows, the more oxygen can flow to your organs. But when your health care practitioner tells you to "exercise" or to take up "aerobic exercise" he or she is not referring solely to "increasing oxygen," but to exercising the heart muscle. The faster it beats, the better a workout it gets (although you don't want to overwork your heart, either).

An exercise is considered aerobic if it makes your heart beat faster than it normally does. When your heart is beating fast, you'll be breathing hard and sweating and will officially be in your "target zone" or "ideal range" (the kind of phrases that turn many people off).

There are official calculations you can make to find this target range. For example, it's recommended that by subtracting your age from 220, then multiplying that number by 60 per cent, you will find your "threshold level"—which means "Your heart should be beating X beats per minute for 20 to 30 minutes." If you multiply the number by 75 per cent, you will find your "ceiling level"—which means "Your heart should not be beating faster than X beats per minute for 20 to 30 minutes." But this is only an example. If you are on heart medications (drugs that slow your heart down, known as beta-blockers), make sure you discuss what "target" to aim for with your health professional.

improving oxygen flow

When more oxygen is in our bodies, we burn fat (see below), our breathing improves, our blood pressure improves, and our hearts work better, which benefits our entire body, leading to regularity, for example. Oxygen also lowers triglycerides and cholesterol, increasing our HDL or "good" cholesterol, while decreasing our LDL or "bad" cholesterol. This means that your arteries will unclog and you may significantly decrease your risk of heart disease and stroke. More oxygen makes our brains work better, so we feel better. Studies show that depression is decreased when we increase oxygen flow into our bodies. Ancient techniques such as yoga, which specifically improve mental and spiritual well-being, achieve this by combining deep breathing and stretching, which improves oxygen and blood flow to specific parts of the body.

Exercise has been shown to dramatically decrease the incidence of many other diseases, including cancer. Some research suggests that cancer cells tend to thrive in an oxygen-depleted environment. The more oxygen in the bloodstream, the less hospitable you make your body to cancer. In addition, since many cancers are related to fat-soluble toxins, the less fat on your body, the less fat-soluble toxins your body can accumulate.

The only kind of exercise that will burn fat is aerobic exercise because *oxygen burns fat*. If you were to go to your fridge and pull out some animal fat (chicken skin, red-meat fat, or butter), throw it in the sink and light it with a match, it will burn. What makes the flame yellow is oxygen; what fuels the fire is the fat. That same process goes on in your body. The oxygen will burn your fat, however you increase the oxygen flow in your body through jumping around, increasing heart rate or employing an established deep-breathing technique.

You can increase the flow of oxygen into your bloodstream without exercising your heart muscle by learning how to breathe deeply through your diaphragm. There are many yoga-like programs (postures, breathing) and videos available that can teach you this technique, which do not require you to jump around. Deep-breathing exercises increase oxygen flow into your bloodstream and can also help to strengthen digestion and keep you regular.

finding your pulse

You have pulse points all over your body. The easiest ones to find are those on your neck, at the base of your thumb, just below your earlobe, or on your wrist. To check your heart rate, look at a watch or clock and begin to count your beats for 15 seconds (if the second hand is on the 12, count until it reaches 15). Then multiply by 4 to get your pulse.

the borg rate of perceived exertion (RPE)

RPE is a way of measuring exercise intensity without finding your pulse, and because of its simplicity, is now the recommended method for judging exertion. The Borg "scale," as it's dubbed, goes from 6–20. An extremely light activity may rate a 7, for example, while a very, very hard activity may rate a 19. Exercise practitioners recommend that you do a "talk test" to rate your exertion, too. If you can't talk without gasping for air, you may be working too hard. You should be able to carry on a normal conversation throughout your activity. What's crucial to remember about RPE is that it is extremely individual; what one person judges a 7, another may judge a 10.

SUGGESTED ACTIVITIES

More Intense	Less Intense
Skiing	Golf
Running	Bowling
Jogging	Badminton
Stair-stepping or Stair-climbing	Croquet
Trampolining	Sailing
Jumping rope	Swimming
Fitness walking	Strolling
Race walking	Stretching
Aerobic classes	
Roller skating	
Ice skating	
Biking	
Weight-bearing exercises	
Tennis	
Swimming	

Note: Certain activities, such as wrestling or weightlifting, are usually of short duration but very intense. As a result, people with certain health problems may not be able to participate in them. For example, if you have heart problems, diabetes, or are taking medications that can affect your heart, intense exercise is not recommended.

Source: Courtesy, Karen Kaye, LPN, A.F.F.A., fitness practitioner

variations on jogging

After warming up with a 15-minute walk, simply walk quickly with maximum exertion for two minutes, then slow down for one minute. Keep your heart rate up on the downhill portion of a walk or a hike by adding lunges or squats.

Vary the way you walk for coordination and balance. Try lifting the knees as high as you can, as if marching. Alternate with a shuffle, letting the tips of your fingers touch the ground as you walk. Do a sideways crab walk. To strengthen the rarely used muscles of the ankles and feet, walk first on the outsides, then on the insides, of your feet. Or practice walking backward.

Use a curb for a step workout. Or climb stairs two at a time.

water workouts

Start by walking in water that's relatively shallow, waist- or chest-deep. Your breathing and heartbeat will determine how hard you are working. Since you'll be moving fairly slowly, pay attention to your body.

For all-over leg toning, take 50 steps forward, 50 steps sideways in crab-like fashion, 50 steps backward, then 50 steps to the other side.

To tone your arms, submerge yourself from the neck down, bringing the arms in and out as if you are clapping. The water will provide natural resistance here.

Deep-water workouts are the most difficult because every move you make is met with resistance. Wear a flotation vest and run without touching the bottom for optimum exertion and little or no impact.

You may also want to try buoyant ankle cuffs and Styrofoam dumbbells or kickboards for full-body conditioning in the water.

deep breathing

Deep relaxation and yoga breathing, such as alternate nostril breath, calms the sympathetic nervous system, thus relaxing the small arteries, and permanently lowers blood pressure.

three

weighty issues

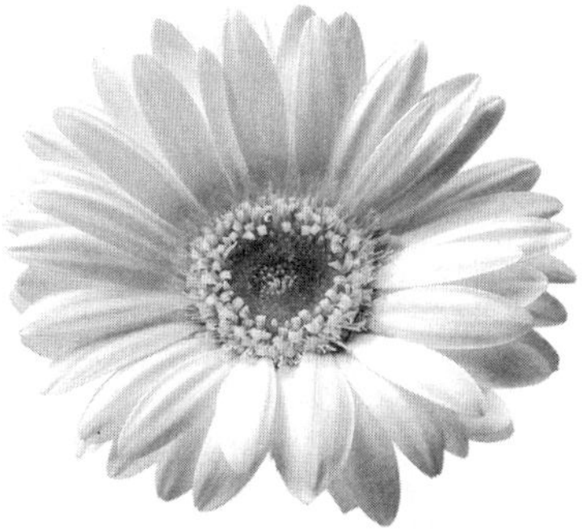

Whether you're underweight or overweight, there are consequences. This chapter focuses on the health risks in women age 50 and over that are associated with obesity and eating disorders. It also exposes some of the myths behind dieting, and some of the psychological reasons for weight gain. What to Eat exposes what's *really* behind the labels and claims of low-fat products, as well as fake fats and sweeteners; it also suggests herbs that improve your ability to digest food. How To Move features postures and stretches that improve digestion, as well as ways to become more active.

weight gain

The best ally you can have on your menopausal journey is 10 extra pounds. I know you don't want to hear this. I understand how difficult it is to desire 10 extra pounds, or to accept those pounds happening to you, as they do to most menopausal women. The North American male-dominant culture's insistence on "beauty equals thin" makes the diet industry a tremendous money-maker.

When thin and young is the standard of beauty, the menopausal woman finds it difficult to maintain a positive self-image as she sees herself transforming into a thick-waisted, silver-haired old woman.

Nonetheless, 10 extra pounds may be your best ally, and I'm not talking 10 pounds of pure fat. You want 10 pounds of fat supported by muscle and bone. And you want to gain that 10 pounds very slowly, about a pound a year after the age of 40, so you'll be in shape for the intense part of your menopausal journey, around 50.

unpacking obesity

At least 80 per cent of women at risk for cardiovascular problems weigh 20 per cent more than they should for their height and age—the technical definition of "obese." When overweight or obese women go to their doctors or nutritionists, they are given meal plans, lists of what and what not to eat, and so on. The problem, however, goes much deeper than simply eating too much food. The key to losing weight for many women is to examine *why* they became obese to begin with.

Obesity is the strongest risk factor for developing cardiovascular problems, common over-50 cancers, such as colon or breast cancer, as well as Type 2 diabetes. Basically, the longer you've been obese, the more you are at risk. Amazingly, experts have noted that when you lose just five pounds, your body actually begins to work more efficiently. But the sentence "eat sensibly and exercise" just doesn't hold any weight for most women battling *theirs.* Part of the story of Western obesity is understanding where the modern diet came from. After all, you didn't create the modern diet; you were born into it. In fact, the root word of "diet" comes from the Greek "*diatta*," meaning "way of life."

a sign of good times

Many European countries experienced a significant drop in a number of obesity-related diseases during the First and Second World Wars, when meat, dairy food, and eggs became scarce in large populations. Wartime rations forced people to survive on brown bread, oats and barley meal and home-grown produce.

Had it not been for the Depression, we may indeed have seen an increase in obesity-related health in North America much earlier than we did. The seeds of sedentary life were already planted in the 1920s, as consumer comforts, mainly the automobile and radio, led to more driving, less walking, and more sedentary recreation. The Depression interrupted what was supposed to be prosperous times for everyone. It also intercepted obesity and all diseases related to obesity, as most industrialized nations barely ate enough to survive.

The Depression years, which ended in Canada when Britain declared war on Germany in 1939, combined with six long years of war, led to an unprecedented yearning for consumer goods such as cars, refrigerators, stoves, radios, and washing machines. As the boys marched home, they were welcomed with open arms into civilian bliss. By 1948, university enrolment had doubled in a decade, leading to an explosion in desk jobs and the commuter economy that exists today. The return of the veterans led to an unprecedented baby boom (your generation), driving the candy, sweets, and junk-food markets for decades to come. Moreover, a sudden influx of money from Victory Bond investments and veterans' re-establishment grants coincided with the first payments of government pensions and family allowances. Never before had North Americans had so much money.

Manufacturers and packaged-goods companies were looking for better ways to compete and sell their products. The answer to their prayers arrived in the late 1940s with the cathode ray tube: television. In the end, television would become the appliance most responsible for dietary decline and sedentary lifestyle as it turned into a babysitter that could mesmerize the baby boom generation for hours.

the diet of leisure

Naturally, after the Second World War, people wanted to celebrate. They gave parties, they drank wine. They smoked. They went to restaurants. More than ever before, our diets began to include more high-fat items, refined carbohydrates, sugar, alcohol, and chemical additives. As women began to manage large families, easy-fix meals in boxes and cans were being manufactured in abundance and sold on television to millions.

The demand for the diet of leisure radically changed agriculture, too. Today, 80 per cent of our grain harvest goes to feed livestock. The rest of our arable land is used for other cash crops such as tomatoes, sugar, coffee, and bananas. Ultimately, cash crops have helped to create the modern Western diet: an obscene amount of meat, eggs, dairy products, sugar, and refined flour.

Since 1940, the use of chemical additives and preservatives in food has risen by 995 per cent. In 1959, the Flavour and Extract Manufacturers Association of the United States (FEMA) established a panel of experts to determine the safety status of food flavourings to deal with the overwhelming number of chemicals that companies wanted to add to foods.

One of the most popular food additives is monosodium glutamate (MSG), the sodium salt of glutamic acid, an amino acid that occurs naturally in protein-containing foods such as meat, fish, milk, and many vegetables. MSG is a flavour enhancer that researchers believe contributes a "fifth taste" to savoury foods such as meats, stews, tomatoes, and cheese.

MSG was originally extracted from seaweed and other plant sources to function in foods the same way as other spices or extracts. Today, MSG is made from starch, corn sugar, or molasses from sugar cane or sugar beets. MSG is produced by a fermentation process similar to that used for making products such as beer, vinegar, and yogurt. While MSG is labelled Generally Recommended As Safe (GRAS) by the United States Food and Drug Administration (FDA), questions about the safety of ingesting MSG have been raised because food sensitivities to the substance have been reported. This fact notwithstanding, the main problem with MSG is that it arouses our appetites even more. Widespread in our food supply, MSG makes food taste better. And the better food tastes, the more we eat.

Hydrolyzed proteins are also used as flavour enhancers. These are made by using enzymes to chemically digest proteins from soy meal, wheat gluten, corn gluten, edible strains of yeast, or other food sources. This process, known as hydrolysis, breaks down proteins into their component amino acids. Today, there are several hundred additive substances like these used in our food, including sugar, baking soda, and vitamins.

Of course, one of the key functions of food additives is to preserve foods for transport. The problem is, once we begin to eat foods that are not indigenous, it loses many of its nutrient properties. Refrigerators make it possible for us to eat tropical foods in Canada and Texas-raised beef in Japan. As a result, few industrialized countries eat indigenously anymore.

minimum wage, maximum fat

The legacy of the Western diet of leisure is that it has become cheaper to eat out of a box or can than off the land. In the developed Western world, where there is minimum wage, there is also maximum fat. At one time, fat was a sign of prosperity and wealth. Today, wealth is defined by thinness and fitness. Ironically, low-fat foods, diet programs, and fitness clubs attract the segment of our population least affected by obesity. In fact, eating disorders tend to plague women who live in higher income brackets.

In 1997, the Coalition for Excess Weight Risk Education, a Washington-based organization comprising the American Diabetes Association, the American Association of Diabetes Educators, the American Society for Clinical Nutrition, the North American Association for the Study of Obesity and four pharmaceutical manufacturers, issued statistics on obesity in the United States. The data can be used to interpret obesity patterns throughout the Western world. Based on a 33-city survey, the National Weight Report found that cities with high unemployment rates and low per capita income tended to have higher rates of obesity. Areas with high annual precipitation rates and a high number of food stores also contributed to obesity. (More rainy or snowy days leads to more snacking in front of the television set!)

why we like our fat

Fat tastes good. Fat also *feels* good in our mouths. Foods that have the particular texture and taste of fat are more acceptable than foods that don't. This is why packaged-foods manufacturers describe their products as "smooth, creamy, moist, tender, and rich." All the foods that boast these qualities, from ice cream or chocolate, to cheese, give us that unique feeling of satiety and satisfaction that makes us feel good.

Eating is a sensual experience. When we enjoy our food, our brains produce endorphins, "feel good" hormones that are, ironically, also produced when we exercise. Eating fat is analogous to having a "mouth orgasm." To many of us, without the taste and texture of fat, eating is an empty experience. And when we're in emotional pain or need, the texture and taste of fat becomes even more important. Bingeing or falling off the diet wagon is not due to "losing control" but to regaining lost "good feelings." Food, as millions of overeaters will tell you, is our friend. It's always there; it never lets us down.

the impact of "low-fat" products

Since the late 1970s, North Americans have been deluged with low-fat products. In 1990, the United States government launched Healthy People 2000, a campaign to urge manufacturers to double their output of low-fat products by the year 2000. Since 1990, more than a thousand new fat-free or low-fat products have been introduced into North American supermarkets annually.

Current guidelines tell us that we should consume less than 30 per cent of calories from fat, while no more than one-third of fat calories should come from saturated fat. According to U.S. estimates, the average person gets between 34–37 per cent of calories from fat and roughly 12 per cent of all calories from saturated fat. Data shows that in terms of "absolute fat," the intake has increased from 81 grams per day in 1980 to 83 grams per day in the 1990s. Total calorie intake has also increased from 1,989 per day in 1980 to 2,153 calories per day. In fact, the only reason that this data shows a drop in the percentage of calories from fat is because of the huge increase in calories consumed per day. The result is that we weigh more today than in 1980, despite the fact that roughly 10,000 more low-fat foods are available to us now than in 1980.

Most of these low-fat products, however, actually encourage us to eat more. For example, if a bag of regular chips has 9 grams of fat per serving (1 serving usually equals about 5 chips or one handful), you will more likely stick to that one handful. However, if you find a low-fat brand of chips that boasts "50 per cent less fat" per serving, you're more likely to eat the whole bag (feeling good about eating "low-fat" chips), which can easily triple your fat intake.

Low-fat or fat-free foods trick our bodies with ingredients that mimic the functions of fat in foods. This effect is often achieved by using modified fats that are only partially metabolized, if at all. While some foods reduce the fat by removing the fat (skim milk, lean cuts of meat), most low-fat foods require a variety of "fat copycats" to preserve the taste and texture of the food. Water, for example, is often combined with carbohydrates and protein to mimic a particular texture or taste, as is the case with a variety of baked goods or cake mixes. In general, though, the low-fat "copycats" are carbohydrate-based, protein-based, or fat-based.

Carbohydrate-based ingredients are starches and gums that are often used as thickening agents to create the texture of fat. You'll find these in abundance in low-fat salad dressings, sauces, gravies, frozen desserts, and baked goods. Compared to natural fats, which are at about 9 calories per gram, carbohydrate-based ingredients run anywhere from zero to 4 calories per gram.

Protein-based, low-fat ingredients are created by "doing things" to the proteins that make them behave differently. For example, by taking proteins such as whey or egg white, and heating or blending them at high speeds, you can create the look and feel of "creamy." Soy and corn proteins are often used in these cases. You'll find these ingredients in low-fat cheese, butter, mayonnaise, salad dressings, frozen dairy desserts, sour cream and baked goods. These items run between 1–4 calories per gram.

Low-fat foods that use fat-based ingredients tailor the fat in some way so that we do not absorb or metabolize it fully. These ingredients are found in chocolate, chocolate coatings, margarine, spreads, sour cream, and cheese. You can also use these ingredients as low-fat substitutes for frying foods (you do this when you fry eggs in margarine, for example). Olestra, the new fat substitute approved by the FDA for use in snack foods only, is an example of a fat substitute that is not absorbed by our bodies, providing no calories. (See page 81 for more detail on olestra.) Caprenin and salatrim are examples of partially absorbed fats (they contain more long-chain fatty acids; see glossary), and are the more traditional fat-based, low-fat ingredients. These contain roughly 5 calories per gram.

There's no question that low-fat foods are designed to give you more freedom of choice with your diet, supposedly allowing you to cut your fat without compromising your taste buds. Studies show that taste outperforms nutrition in your brain. Yet, many experts believe that low-fat products create more of a barrier to weight loss in the long term. Researchers at the University of Toronto suggest that these products essentially allow us to increase our calories even though we are reducing our overall fat intake. For example, in one study, women who consumed a low-fat breakfast food ate more during the day than women who consumed a higher-fat food at breakfast.

The good news about low-fat or fat-free products is that they are, in fact, lower in fat, and are created to substitute for the "bad foods" you know you shouldn't have but "cannot live without." The boring phrase "everything in moderation" applies to low-fat products, too. Balancing these products with good stuff is the key. A low-fat treat should still be treated like its high-fat original. In other words, don't have double the amount because it's low-fat. Instead, have the same amount as you would of the original.

chronic dieting

The road to obesity is paved with chronic dieting. Indeed, many women say that they've "dieted themselves up" to their present wieght. It is estimated that at least 50 per cent of all North American women are dieting at any given time, while one-third of North American dieters initiate a diet at least once a month. The very act of dieting in your teens and 20s can predispose you to obesity later in life. This occurs because most people "crash and burn" instead of eating sensibly. In other words, they're chronic dieters.

The crash-and-burn approach to diet is do when we want to lose a specific number of pounds for a particular occasion or outfit. The pattern is to starve for a few days and then eat normally. Or, we eat only certain foods (like celery and grapefruit) for a number of days and then eat normally after we've lost the weight. Most of these diets do not incorporate exercise, which means that we burn up some of our muscle as well as fat. Then, when we eat normally, we gain only fat. And over the years, that fat simply grows fatter. The bottom line is that when there is more fat on your body than muscle, you cannot burn calories as efficiently. It is the muscle that makes it possible to burn calories. Diet it away, and you diet away your ability to burn fat.

If starvation is involved in our trying to lose weight, our bodies become more efficient at getting fat. Starvation triggers an intelligence in the metabolism; our body suddenly thinks we're living in a war zone and goes into super-efficient nomadic mode, not realizing that we're living in North America. So, when we return to our normal caloric intake, or even a lower-than-normal caloric intake after we've starved ourselves, *we gain more weight*. Our bodies say: "Oh look—food! Better store that as fat for the next famine." Some researchers believe that starvation diets slow down our metabolic rates far below normal so that weight gain becomes more rapid after each starvation episode.

This cycle of crash or starvation dieting is known as the yo-yo diet syndrome, the subject of thousands of articles in women's magazines throughout the last 20 years. Breaking the pattern sounds easy: combine exercise with a sensible diet. But it's not that easy if you've led a sedentary life most of your adult years. Ninety-five per cent of the people who go on a diet gain back the weight they lost, as well as extra weight, within two years. As discussed further on, the failure often lies in psychological and behavioural factors. We have to understand why we need to eat before we can eat less. The best way to break the yo-yo diet pattern is to educate your children early about food habits and appropriate body weight. Experts say that unless you are significantly overweight to begin with or have a medical condition, *don't diet*.

biological causes of obesity

Eating too much high-fat or high-calorie food while remaining sedentary is certainly one biological cause of obesity. Furthermore, a woman's metabolism slows down by 25 per cent after menopause, which means that unless she either decreases her calories by 25 per cent or increases her activity level by 25 per cent, to compensate, she will probably gain weight. There are also other hormonal problems that contribute to obesity, such as an underactive thyroid gland (hypothyroidism), which is very common in women over 50.

Since making diet and lifestyle changes is so difficult, however, there is an interest in finding genetic causes for obesity. A genetic cause would mean that obesity is beyond our control, something we've inherited, a notion which would probably be comforting for many people. Researchers active in the Human Genome Project, a project that intends to map every gene in the human body, are actively looking for the "obesity gene" or "fat gene." But few scientists believe that obesity is simply genetic. In other words, there are so many environmental and social factors that can trip the obesity switch, finding a specific gene for obesity is about as worthwhile as finding the "anger gene" or "crime gene."

some theories

An important theory about why we get fat focuses on insulin resistance. It's believed that when the body produces too much insulin, we eat more to try to maintain a balance. This is why weight gain is often the first symptom of Type 2 diabetes. But then we have to ask what causes insulin resistance to begin with; and many researchers believe that it is triggered by obesity. So it becomes a chicken-or-egg puzzle.

There are also many theories surrounding the function of fat cells. Are some people genetically programmed to have more, or "fatter," fat cells than others? No answers here yet.

What about the brain and obesity? Some researchers propose that obesity is "all in the head." That is, it somehow malfunctions when it comes to sending the message "I'm full." It's believed that the hypothalamus, a part of the brain that controls messages to other parts of the body, may control "satiation messages."

what about the fat hormone?

A study reported in a 1997 issue of *Nature Medicine* showed that people with low levels of the hormone leptin may be prone to weight gain. In this study, people who gained an average of 50 pounds over three years started out with lower leptin levels than people who maintained their weight over the same period. Therefore, this study may form the basis for treating obesity with leptin.

Experts speculate that 10 per cent of all obesity may be due to leptin resistance. Leptin is made by fat cells and apparently sends messages to the brain about how much fat our bodies are carrying. Like other hormones, it's thought that leptin has a stimulating action that acts as a thermostat of sorts. In mice, adequate amounts of leptin somehow signalled the mouse to become more active and eat less, while too little leptin signalled the mouse to eat more while becoming less active.

Interestingly, the Pima Indians of southern Arizona and northern New Mexico, who are prone to obesity, were shown to have roughly one-third less leptin in blood analyses. Human studies of injecting leptin to treat obesity are in the works right now, but to date have not been shown to be effective.

drug treatment for obesity

Drug treatment for obesity has an awfully shady history. Women have been abused repeatedly by the medical system. Throughout the 1950s, 1960s, and as late as the 1970s, women were prescribed thyroxine, which is thyroid hormone, to speed up their metabolisms. Unless a person has an underactive thyroid gland, or no thyroid gland (which may have been surgically removed), this is a very dangerous medication, which can cause heart failure. Request a thyroid function test before you accept this medication.

Amphetamines or "speed" were often widely peddled to women as well by doctors, but they too are dangerous, and can put your health at risk.

anti-obesity pills

The U.S. government recently approved an anti-obesity pill that blocks the absorption of almost one-third of the fat people eat. One of the side effects of this new prescription drug, called orlistat (Xenical®), causes rather embarrassing diarrhea each time you eat fatty foods. To avoid the drug's side effects, simply avoid fat! The pill can also decrease absorption of vitamin D and other important nutrients.

Now available in Canada, orlistat is the first drug to fight obesity through the intestine instead of the brain. Taken with each meal, it binds to certain pancreatic enzymes to block the digestion of 30 per cent of the fat you ingest. How it affects the pancreas in the long term is not known. Combined with a sensible diet, people on orlistat lost more weight than those not on orlistat. This drug is not intended for people who need to lose a few pounds; it is designed for medically obese people. Orlistat was also found to lower cholesterol, blood pressure, and blood sugar levels.

Another obesity pill, called Redux®, alters brain chemicals to trick the body into feeling full. A similar competitor, sibutramine, is expected to be approved by the end of 1998.

One of the most controversial anti-obesity therapies was the use of fenfluramine and phentermine (Fen/Phen). Both drugs were approved for use individually more than 20 years ago, but since 1992, doctors tended to prescribe them together for long-term management of obesity. In 1996, U.S. doctors wrote a total of 18 million monthly prescriptions for Fen/Phen. Many of these prescriptions were issued to people who were not obese. This is known as off-label prescribing. In July 1997, the FDA, and researchers at the Mayo Clinic and the Mayo Foundation made a joint announcement warning doctors that Fen/Phen can cause heart disease. On September 15, 1997, "Fen" was taken off the market. The Fen/Phen lesson: diet and lifestyle modification are still the best pathways to wellness. More bad news has surfaced about Fen/Phen wreaking havoc on serotonic levels, which only reinforces the message.

eating disorders

For 2 per cent of the female population in North America, starving and purging are considered a normal way to control weight. Only a small portion of women are obese because of truly hereditary factors. Most women who think they are overweight are, in fact, at an *ideal* weight for their height and body size.

In Western society, the fear of obesity is so crippling that 60 per cent of young girls develop distorted body images between grades one and six, believing that they are fat; 70 per cent of all women begin dieting between the ages of 14 and 21. A U.S. study of high-school girls found that 53 per cent were unhappy with their bodies by age 13; and by age 18, 78 per cent were dissatisfied. The most disturbing fact, revealed in the 1991 critically acclaimed Canadian documentary *The Famine Within*, is that when given a choice, most women *would rather be dead than fat*! Eating disorders are so widespread that abnormal patterns of eating are increasingly accepted in the general population. There are parents who are actually *starving* their young daughters in an effort to keep them thin.

The two most common eating disorders involve starvation. They are *anorexia nervosa* ("loss of appetite due to mental disorder"), and bingeing followed by purging, known as *bulimia nervosa* ("hunger like an ox due to mental disorder"). Women will purge after a bingeing episode by inducing vomiting, abusing laxatives, diuretics, and thyroid hormone. The most horrifying examples occur in women with Type 1 diabetes who sometimes deliberately withhold their insulin to control their weight.

Perhaps the most accepted weight-control behaviour is overexercising. Today, rigorous, strenuous exercise is used as a method of "purging," and has become one of the tenets of socially accepted feminine behaviour. A skeleton with biceps is the current ideal.

Women with a history of eating disorders are at much greater risk of developing osteoporosis. Women who are carrying a bit of weight have stronger bones than thin women. Osteoporosis is even on the rise in anorexic women as young as 20.

why do we do this?

Eating disorders are diseases of control that primarily affect women, although more men are becoming vulnerable in recent years. Bulimics and anorexics are usually overachievers in other aspects of their lives, and view excess weight as an announcement to the world that they are "out of control." This view becomes more distorted as time goes on, until the act of eating food in public (in bulimia) or at all (in anorexia) is equivalent to a loss of control.

In anorexia, the person's emotional and sensual desires are perceived through food. These unmet desires are so great that the anorexic fears that once she eats she'll never stop since her appetite will know no natural boundaries; the fear of food drives the disease.

Most of us find it easier to relate to the bulimic than the anorexic; bulimics express their loss of control through bingeing in the same way that others may yell at their children. Bulimics then purge to regain their control. There is a feeling of comfort for bulimics in both the binge and the purge. Bulimics are sometimes referred to as "failed anorexics" because they'd starve if they could. Anorexics, however, are masters of control. They never break. I once asked a recovering anorexic the dumb question, "But didn't you get *hungry*?" Her response was that the hunger pangs made her feel powerful. The more intense the hunger, the more powerful she felt; the power actually gave her a "high."

compulsive eating disorders

When we hear "eating disorder," we usually think about anorexia or bulimia. There are many people, however, who binge without purging. This is also known as binge eating disorder (a.k.a. compulsive overeating). In this case, the bingeing is still an announcement to the world that "I'm out of control." Someone who purges is hiding a lack of control. Someone who binges and never purges is *advertising* a lack of control. The purger is passively asking for help; the binger who doesn't purge is aggressively asking for help. It's the same disease with a different result.

There is one more layer when it comes to compulsive overeating, which is considered to be controversial, and often rejected by the overeater: the desire to get fat is often behind the compulsion. Many people who overeat insist that fat is a consequence of eating food, not a *goal*. Many therapists who deal with overeating disagree, and believe that if a woman admits that she has an emotional interest in actually being large, she may be much closer to stopping her compulsion to eat. Furthermore, many women who eat compulsively do not recognize that they are doing so.

Profile of a Compulsive Eater

- Eating when you're not hungry
- Feeling out of control when you're around food, either trying to resist it or gorging on it
- Spending a lot of time thinking or worrying about food and weight
- Always desperate to try another diet that promises results
- Feelings of self-loathing and shame
- Hating your own body
- Obsessed with what you can or will eat, or have eaten
- Eating in secret or with "eating friends"
- Appearing in public to be a professional dieter who's in control

- Buying cakes or pies as "gifts" and having them wrapped to hide the fact that they're for you
- Having a pristine kitchen with only the "right" foods
- Feeling either out-of-control with food (compulsive eating), or imprisoned by it (dieting)
- Feeling temporary relief by not eating
- Looking forward with pleasure and anticipation to the time when you can eat alone
- Feeling unhappy because of your eating behaviour

the issue of hunger

Most people eat when they're hungry. But if you're a compulsive eater, hunger cues have nothing to do with when you eat. You may eat for any of the following reasons:

1. Eating as a social event: this includes family meals, or meeting friends at restaurants. The point is that you plan food as the social entertainment. Most of us do this, but often we do it when we're not even hungry.
2. Eating to satisfy "mouth hunger"—the need to have something in your mouth, even though you are not hungry.
3. Eating to prevent future hunger: "Better eat now because later I may not get a chance."
4. Eating as a reward for a bad day or bad experience; or to reward yourself for a good day or good experience.
5. Eating because "It's the only pleasure I can count on!"
6. Eating to quell nerves.
7. Eating because you're bored.
8. Eating now because you're "going on a diet" tomorrow. (Hence, the eating is done out of a real fear that you will be deprived later.)
9. Eating because food is your friend.

12 steps to change

Food addiction, like other addictions, can be treated successfully with a 12-step program. For those of you who aren't familiar with this type of program, I've provided the text of "The 12 Steps" in Table 3.1.

The 12-step program was started in the 1930s by an alcoholic who was able to overcome his addiction by essentially saying, "God, help me!" He found other alcoholics who were in a similar position, and through an organized, nonjudgmental support system, they overcame their addiction by realizing that "God" (a higher power, spirit, force, physical properties of the universe or intelligence) *helps those who help themselves*. In other words, you have to want the help. This is the premise of Alcoholics Anonymous, the most successful recovery program for addicts that exists.

People with other addictions have adopted the same program, using Alcoholics Anonymous and the "The 12 Steps and 12 Traditions," the founding literature for Alcoholics Anonymous. Overeaters Anonymous (OA) substitutes the phrase "compulsive overeater" for "alcoholic," and "food" for "alcohol." The theme of all 12-step programs is best expressed through the Serenity Prayer, the first line being "God grant me the serenity to accept the things I cannot change; change the things I can, and the wisdom to know the difference." In other words, you can't take back the food you ate yesterday or last year but you can control the food you eat today instead of feeling guilty about yesterday.

Every 12-step program also contains the 12 Traditions, which, essentially, is a code of conduct. To join an OA program, you need only to take the first step. Abstinence and the next two steps is what most people are able to do in a 6–12 month period before moving on. In an OA program, "abstinence" means three meals daily, weighed and measured, with nothing in between except sugar-free or no-calorie beverages, and sugar-free gum. Your food is written down and called in. The program also advises you to obtain your doctor's approval before starting. Abstinence is continued through a continuous process of one-day-at-a-time and "sponsors"—people who call you to check in, and who you can call when the cravings hit. Sponsors are recovering overeaters who have been there and who can talk you through your cravings.

OA membership is predominantly female; if you are interested in joining OA and are male, you may feel more comfortable in an all-male group. Many women overeaters overeat because they have been harmed by men, and their anger is often directed at the one male in the room; this may not be a comfortable position if you're a male overeater. For this reason, OA is divided into all-female and all-male groups.

TABLE 3.1: THE 12 STEPS OF OVEREATERS ANONYMOUS

Step One: I admit I am powerless over food and that my life has become unmanageable.
Step Two: I've come to believe that a Power greater than myself can restore me to sanity.
Step Three: I've made a decision to turn my will and my life over to the care of a Higher Power, as I understand it.
Step Four: I've made a searching and fearless moral inventory of myself.
Step Five: I've admitted to a Higher Power, to myself, and to another human being the exact nature of my wrongs.
Step Six: I'm entirely ready to have a Higher Power remove all these defects of character.
Step Seven: I've humbly asked a Higher Power to remove my shortcomings.
Step Eight: I've made a list of all persons I have harmed and have become willing to make amends to them all.
Step Nine: I've made direct amends to such people wherever possible, except when to do so would injure them or others.
Step Ten: I've continued to take personal inventory and when I was wrong, promptly admitted it.
Step Eleven: I've sought through prayer and meditation to improve my conscious contact with a Higher Power, as I understand it, praying only for knowledge of Its will for me and the power to carry that out.
Step Twelve: Having had a spiritual awakening as the result of these steps, I've tried to carry this message to compulsive overeaters and to practice these principles in all my affairs.

Source: Overeaters Anonymous, 1997.

what to eat

Variety is the key to a healthy diet. If your meal contains mostly carbohydrates (50–55 per cent), some protein (15–20 per cent), not much fat (less than 30 per cent), and limited sugar, you're eating well.

Imagine yourself in a supermarket with a shopping cart. What you need to live is usually found on the *outside* aisles of any supermarket or grocery store. Outside aisles simulate the foods you can buy at outdoor markets:

fruits, vegetables, meat, eggs, fish, breads, and dairy products. Natural fibre, both soluble and insoluble, is also found in the outside aisles. But remember: foods you buy in the outside aisles can also be high in fat unless you select wisely.

reading food labels

The inside aisles of a supermarkets are not only the aisles of temptation, they may contain products with complicated food labels. In Canada, ingredients on labels are listed according to weight, with the "most" listed first. If sugar is the first ingredient, you know the product contains mostly sugar. The lower the sugar appears on the list, the less sugar contained in the product. The nutrition information on the label should also list the total amount of carbohydrates in a serving of the food. That amount includes both natural and added sugars.

Whenever a product says it is "calorie-reduced" or "carbohydrate-reduced" it means there are 50 per cent less calories or carbohydrates compared to the original product. But something that was originally 7,000 calories isn't much better at 3,500.

"Cholesterol-free" or "low cholesterol" means that the product doesn't have any, or much, animal fat (hence, cholesterol). This doesn't mean "low fat." Pure vegetable oil doesn't come from animals but is pure fat!

A label that screams "low fat" means that the product has less than 3 grams of fat per serving. In potato-chip country, that means about 6 potato chips. I don't know anybody who ever ate one serving of potato chips! So if you eat the whole bag of "low-fat" chips, you're still eating a lot of fat. Be sure to check serving sizes.

Products that are "light" (or "lite") mean that there is 25–50 per cent less of some ingredient in that product. It could be fat, cholesterol, salt, or sugar, or less food colouring, and therefore the designation is frequently misleading.

"sugar-free"

Careful! "Sugar-free" in the language of labels simply means "sucrose-free." That doesn't mean the product is carbohydrate free, as in: dextrose-free, lactose-free, glucose-free, or fructose-free. Check the labels for all things ending in "ose" to find out the sugar content; you're not just looking for sucrose. Watch out for "no added sugar," "without added sugar," or "no sugar added."

This simply means: "We didn't put the sugar in, God did." Again, reading the carbohydrates line on the nutrition information label is the most accurate way to determine the amount of sugar contained in the product. Nutrition claims in big, bold statements can be misleading.

"less and more"

And then there are the "comparison claims" such as "fewer," "reduced," "less," "more," or my favourite—"light". These words appear on foods that have been nutritionally altered from a previous "version" or competitor's version. For example, Brand X Potato Chips—Regular may have much more fat than Brand X Potato Chips—Lite "With less Fat than Regular Brand X " That doesn't mean that Brand X Lite is fat-free, or even, low in fat. It just means it's X per cent *lower* in fat than Brand X Regular.

On the flip side, Brand Y may have a trace amount of calcium, while Brand Y—"now with more calcium"—may still have a small amount of calcium, but 10 per cent more than Brand Y. (In other words, you may still need to eat 100 bowls of Brand Y before you get the daily requirement for calcium!)

To be light or "lite," a product has to contain either one-third fewer calories or half the fat of the regular product. Or, a low-calorie or low-fat food contains 50 per cent less sodium. Something that is "light in sodium" means it has at least 50 per cent less sodium than the regular product, such as canned soup. (But if you're buying hair colour that reads "light brown," "light" is a descriptive word, not referring to an ingredient!)

born in the U.S.A.

American labels that say "sugar-free" contain less than 0.5 grams of sugar per serving, while a "reduced-sugar" food contains at least 25 per cent less sugar per serving than the regular product. If the label also states that the product is not a reduced- or low-calorie food, or it is not meant for weight control, it has enough sugar in there to make you think twice.

Serving sizes in the United States are also listed differently. Foods that are similar are given the same *type* of serving size defined by the FDA. That means that 5 cereals that all weigh X grams per cup will share the same serving sizes.

Calories (how much energy) and calories from fat (how much fat) are also listed per serving of food in the United States. Total carbohydrate, dietary fibre, sugars, other carbohydrates (which means starches), total fat, saturated fat, cholesterol, sodium, potassium, and vitamins and minerals are given in

Percent Daily values, based on the 2,000-calorie diet recommended by the U.S. government. In Canada, Recommended Nutrient Intake (RNI) is used for vitamins and minerals.

fake fat

We have artificial sweeteners; why not artificial fat? This question has led to the creation of an emerging yet highly suspicious ingredient: fat substitutes, designed to replace real fat and hence reduce the calories from real fat without compromising the taste. This is done by creating a fake fat that the body cannot absorb.

One of the first fat substitutes was Simplesse, an All-Natural Fat Substitute, made from milk and egg-white protein, which was developed by the NutraSweet Company. Simplesse apparently adds 1–2 calories per gram instead of the usual 9 calories per gram from fat. Other fat substitutes simply take protein and carbohydrates and modify them in some way to simulate the textures of fat (creamy, smooth, and so on). All of these fat substitutes help to create low-fat products.

The calorie-free fat substitute olestra was developed by Procter & Gamble Inc., and is currently being test marketed in the United States in a variety of savoury snacks such as potato chips and crackers. Olestra is a potentially dangerous ingredient that most experts feel can do more harm than good. Canada has not yet approved it.

Olestra is made from a combination of vegetable oils and sugar. Therefore, it tastes just like the real thing, but the biochemical structure is a molecule too big for the liver to break down. So, olestra just gets passed into the large intestine and is excreted. Olestra is more than an "empty" molecule, however. According to the FDA Commissioner of Food and Drugs, olestra may cause diarrhea and cramps and may deplete the body of vital nutrients, including vitamins A, D, E, and K, necessary for blood to clot. Indeed, all studies conducted by Procter & Gamble have shown this potential. If the FDA approves olestra for use as a cooking-oil substitute, you'll see it in every imaginable high-fat product.

There is another danger with olestra, which nutritionists raised in a critique of olestra published in a 1996 issue of the *University of California at Berkeley Wellness Letter*, the year olestra was approved for test markets. The article states that instead of encouraging people to choose nutritious foods, such as fruits, grains, and vegetables over high-fat foods, products like olestra encourage a high *fake*-fat diet that's still too low in fibre and other essential nutrients. And the no-fat icing on the cake is that people who ingest olestra could potentially wind up with a vitamin deficiency, to boot. Products like olestra should make you nervous.

sweeteners

Here's what you need to know about sweeteners if you're trying to cut down on fat. While artificial sweeteners do not contain sugar (for diabetics, this means they will not affect blood sugar levels) they *may* contain a tiny amount of calories. It depends upon whether that sweetener is classified as nutritive or non-nutritive.

Nutritive sweeteners have calories or contain natural sugar. White or brown table sugar, molasses, honey, and syrup are all considered nutritive sweeteners. *Sugar alcohols* are also nutritive sweeteners because they are made from fruits or produced commercially from dextrose. Sorbitol, mannitol, xylitol, and maltitol are all sugar alcohols. Sugar alcohols contain only 4 calories per gram, like ordinary sugar, and will affect blood sugar levels like ordinary sugar. It all depends on how much is consumed, and the degree of absorption from your digestive tract. (See page 84 for more detail on sugar alcohols.)

Non-nutritive sweeteners are sugar substitutes or artificial sweeteners; they do not have any calories and will not affect your blood sugar levels. Examples of non-nutritive sweeteners are saccharin, cyclamate, aspartame, sucralose, and acesulflame potassium.

the sweetener wars

The oldest non-nutritive sweetener is saccharin, which is what you get when you purchase Sweet'n Low® or Hermesetas. In Canada, saccharin can only be used as a tabletop sweetener in either tablet or powder form. Saccharin is 300 times sweeter than sucrose (table sugar) but has a metallic aftertaste. At one point in the 1970s, saccharin was also thought to cause cancer, but this claim was never proven.

In the 1980s, aspartame was invented, which is sold as NutraSweet®. Aspartame is also available as a tabletop sweetener under the brand name Equal®, and most recently, PROSWEET. It was considered a nutritive sweetener because it was derived from natural sources (two amino acids—aspartic acids and phenylalanine), which means that aspartame is digested and metabolized the same way as any other protein foods. For every gram of aspartame, there are 4 calories, but since aspartame is 200 times sweeter than sugar, you don't need very much of it to achieve the desired sweetness.

In at least 90 countries, aspartame is found in more than 150 product categories, including breakfast cereals, beverages, desserts, candy and gum, syrups, salad dressings, and various snack foods.

An interesting point about aspartame is that it's not recommended for baking or any other recipe where heat is required. The two amino acids in this substance separate with heat and the product loses its sweetness. That's not to say it's harmful if heated, but your recipe won't turn out.

For the moment, aspartame is considered safe for everybody, including people with diabetes, pregnant women, and children. The only people who are cautioned against consuming it are those with a rare hereditary disease known as phenylketonuria (PKU), because aspartame contains phenylalanine, which people with PKU cannot tolerate.

Another common tabletop sweetener is sucralose, sold as Splenda. Splenda is a white crystalline powder, actually made from sugar itself. It's 600 times sweeter than table sugar but is not broken down in your digestive system, so it has no calories at all. Splenda can also be used in hot or cold foods, and is found in hot and cold beverages, frozen foods, baked goods, and other packaged foods.

In the United States, you can still purchase cyclamate, a non-nutritive sweetener sold under the brand name Sucaryl or Sugar Twin. Cyclamate is also the sweetener used in many weight-control products and is 30 times sweeter than table sugar, with no aftertaste. Cyclamate can be used in hot or cold foods. In Canada, however, you can only find cyclamate as Sugar Twin or as a sugar substitute in medication.

the newest sweeteners

One of the most recent additions to the sweeteners is acesuflame potassium (Ace-K). About 200 times sweeter than table sugar, Ace-K is sold as Sunett and is found in beverages, fruit spreads, baked goods, dessert bases, tabletop sweeteners, hard candies, chewing gum, and breath fresheners. While no specific studies on Ace-K and diabetes have been done, the only people who are cautioned against ingesting Ace-K are those on a potassium-restricted diet or those who are allergic to sulpha drugs.

sugar alcohols

Not to be confused with alcoholic beverages, sugar alcohols are nutritive sweeteners, like regular sugar. These are found naturally in fruits or manufactured from carbohydrates. Sorbitol, mannitol, xylitol, maltitol, maltitol syrup, lactitol, isomalt, and hydrogenated starch hydrolysates are all sugar alcohols. In your body, these types of sugars are absorbed lower down in the digestive tract, and will cause gastrointestinal symptoms if you use too much.

Because sugar alcohols are absorbed more slowly, they were once touted as ideal for people with diabetes, but since they are a carbohydrate they still increase blood sugar—just like regular sugar. Now that artificial sweeteners are on the market in abundance, the only real advantage of sugar alcohols is that they don't cause cavities. The bacteria in your mouth don't like sugar alcohols as much as real sugar.

According to the FDA, even foods that contain sugar alcohols can be labelled "sugar-free." Sugar alcohol products can also be labelled "Does not promote tooth decay," which is often confused with "low-calorie."

spices good for digestion

- Coriander. Eases gases and works to tone the digestive system. Use powdered or whole-seed, or garnish with fresh leaves (cilantro).
- Cardamom. Reduces the mucus-forming effects of dairy products. Use powdered or whole seeds.
- Turmeric. Improves metabolism and helps you to digest proteins. Use the root ground. (Note: Turmeric gives dishes a yellowish colour and can stain clothes and china.)
- Black pepper. Stimulates appetite and helps you digest dairy products. Use freshly ground.
- Cumin. Helps reduce gases and generally tones the digestive system. Use seeds whole or powdered.
- Fennel. Helps prevent gas. Chew the seeds after eating, or add them to vegetables that tend to produce gas when cooking. Use whole or powdered.
- Ginger. Aids digestion and respiration. Also helps to relieve gas and constipation, or indigestion. Use root fresh or dried. (Note: ginger can aggravate bleeding ulcers.)

- Cinnamon. Naturally cleanses your digestive system. Use powdered, in sticks or pieces.
- Nutmeg. Helps your body absorb nutrients from food, but should be used sparingly.
- Cloves. Helps your body absorb nutrients. Use whole or ground.
- Cayenne. Helps to simulate your digestive juices, and is known for having a cleansing action within the large intestine. Helps to relieve that feeling of fullness after eating a heavy meal.

With the advent of the Internet, "e-dieting" is now becoming a popular pusuit which allows for anonymity and privacy.

Online Dieting

There are a number of commercial diet sites online, such as eDiets.com (Florida-based) or Cyberdiet.com (California-based). Many women are finding this is a good alternative to joining a health club or diet program that requires personal check-ins. Online dieting is a good option if you're looking for the following:

- nutrition, exercise, and motivation
- online chats about dieting or eating disorders
- a computer-generated schedule for weight loss; for example, a 12-week plan, with meal plans and shopping lists, which is adjusted to reflect the diet's progress, reported weekly
- dietitians and psychologists for online consults
- subscription information, such as newsletters
- special menus, personalized depending on what you need to cut down on (sodium, cholesterol, dairy, and so on)

how to move

For a lot of women, just getting up and out is a healthy start. Ideally, adopting a heart-smart exercise program, outlined in chapter 2, is the best way to shed some pounds. But you know what? Exercise practitioners hate the terms "aerobic activity" or "aerobics program" because it is not about what people do in their daily life. Health promoters are replacing these terms with the phrase "active living"—because that's what becoming unsedentary is all about.

There are many ways you can adopt an active lifestyle. Here are some suggestions:

- If you drive everywhere, pick the parking space farther away from your destination so you can work some daily walking into your life.
- If you take public transit everywhere, get off one or two stops early so you can walk the rest of the way to your destination.
- Choose stairs more often over escalators or elevators.
- Park at one side of the mall and then walk to the other.
- Take a stroll after dinner around your neighbourhood.
- Volunteer to walk the dog.
- On weekends, go to the zoo or get out to flea markets, garage sales, and so on.

start slow

Reports from the United States show that one out of three American adults are overweight, a sign of growing inactivity that we're seeing in Canada, too. Some people are so put off by the health club scene, they become even more sedentary. This is similar to diet failure, where you become so demoralized that you "cheated," and binge even more.

What's the definition of sedentary? *Not moving*! If you have a desk job or spend most of your time at a computer, in your car, or watching television (even if it is PBS or CNN), you are a sedentary person. If you do roughly 20 minutes of exercise less than once a week, you're relatively sedentary. You need to incorporate some sort of movement into your daily schedule in order to be considered active. That movement can be anything: aerobic exercise, brisk walks around the block, or walking your dog.

If you've been sedentary most of your life, there's nothing wrong with starting off with simple, even leisurely activities such as gardening, feeding the birds in a park, or doing a few simple stretches. Any step you make towards being more active is a crucial and important one.

A 1998 *New England Journal of Medicine* article reported that low-intensity exercises such as walking were associated with lower rates of a range of health problems, including heart disease (see chapter 2), certain cancers, diabetes (see chapter 7), and depression (see chapter 8).

Experts also recommend that you find a friend, neighbour, or relative to get physical with you. When your exercise plans include someone else, you'll be less apt to cancel acrtivities or make excuses for not getting out there.

prepare for "moving day"

Choose an activity that's right for you. Whether it's walking, chopping wood, jumping rope, or folk dancing, pick something you enjoy. You don't have to do the same thing each time, either. Vary your routine to avoid monotony. Just make sure that whatever activity you choose is continuous for the duration; walking for two minutes then stopping for three isn't continuous. It's also important to choose an activity that doesn't aggravate a pre-existing health problem. Try not to let two days pass without doing something. And pick a duration. If you're elderly or ill, even a few minutes of activity is a good start. If you're sedentary but otherwise healthy, aim for 20 to 30 minutes.

postures that improve digestion

1. Locust: Lie on your belly with your arms folded beneath you, palms pressed in to your body. Extend both legs until they lift up and off the floor. Keep the toes pointed. Release.
2. Cobra (Upward-Facing Dog): Lie on your belly with your palms down and adjacent to your shoulders. Slowly raise your upper body, lifting all but the lower abdomen toward the ceiling. Breathe deeply. Release.
3. Fish: Lie on your back. Place your hands under your sitting bones, palms pressed in to the floor, feet flexed. Gently roll one, then the other shoulder inward, shortening the distance between your shoulder blades (your chest will naturally arch upwards). Breathe, lengthening your abdominals and ribcage (see figure i). Release.

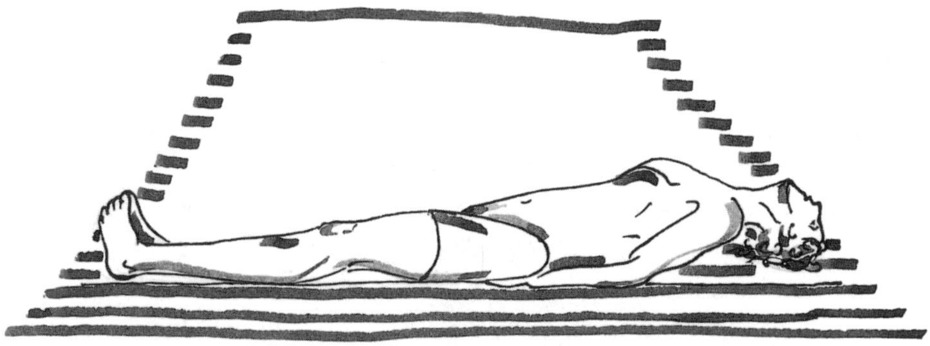

figure i

four

breast health

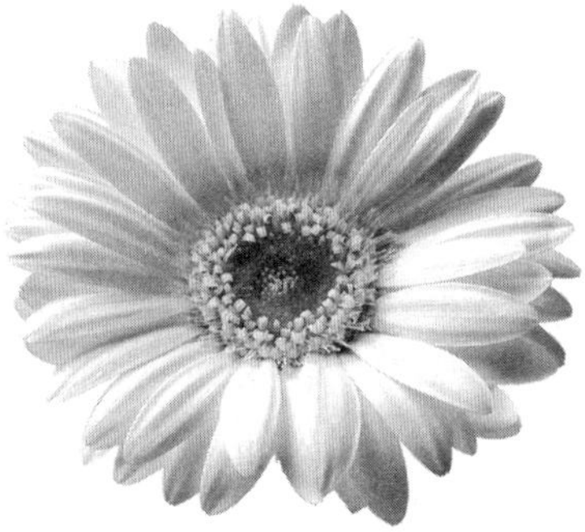

Let's not beat around the bush: the term "breast health" really means "what can I do to avoid breast cancer?" So that's what this chapter is all about. All the latest information on mammography, genetic screening, detection and prevention of breast cancer is here, including information on tamoxifen as a prevention drug. This chapter does not explore breast cancer treatment, which is thoroughly covered in my book, *The Breast Sourcebook*.

reviewing the known risk factors

Seventy per cent of women who develop breast cancer have no known risk factors. Given that statistic, what does it mean when you're told you're "at risk" for breast cancer—or any other disease? A few things, depending on the adjective that precedes the word "risk." The risks you can do something about are considered modifiable risk factors. These are risks that can be reduced, prevented, or altered through behaviour (like quitting smoking or eating a balanced diet). The risks you can't do anything about, such as your age or family history, can still be lowered by eliminating modifiable risk factors. The following "risk list" is arranged alphabetically to make it easier for you to access the information you may want right now.

age

The risk of breast cancer is largely age-related. It's rare to see breast cancer under age 30, less common to see it between the ages of 30–40, and most common in developed nations after menopause (or after age 50). For example, looking at North American statistics from 1984–1988, only 0.9 per 100,000 women were diagnosed with breast cancer in the 20–24 age group compared to 66.2 per 100,000 cases of breast cancer in the 30–34 age group. However, in women 45–49, that number rose to 187.4 per 100,000 women, increased to 220 per 100,000 in the 50–54 age group, leaped up to 390.7 per 100,000 women in the 65–69 age group, and peaked at 461.4 per 100,000 women in the 75–79 age group. The 1 in 8 figure refers to your risk over a lifetime, assuming that you live to 95.

Another way of looking at your age-related risk is to break it down into five-year intervals (assuming American statistics). In this case, by age 30, you have a 1 in 2,525 chance of developing breast cancer; by 35, the figure jumps to 1 in 622; by 40, it rises to 1 in 217; by 45, it's 1 in 93; by 50, 1 in 50; by 55, 1 in 33; by 60, 1 in 24; by 65, 1 in 17; by 70, 1 in 14; by 75, 1 in 11; by 80, 1 in 10; by 85, 1 in 9; and over 85, 1 in 8.

bad habits

Any lifestyle indulgence that has proven risk factors is, for the purpose of this chapter, considered a "bad habit." If you smoke, drink an excessive amount of alcohol, or abuse illegal drugs, your risk of contracting some diseases is higher than for people who don't do these things.

Alcohol and cigarettes have been linked to a variety of cancers; breast cancer is no exception. A 1994 survey conducted by the American Cancer Society suggested that smokers were 25 per cent more likely than non-smokers or ex-smokers to die of breast cancer. This is different than saying "Smoking causes breast cancer," however. It's really saying, "Non-smokers have a better chance of avoiding breast cancer than smokers." It might also mean that smokers who get breast cancer are more likely to die of it. However, smoking does conclusively cause lung cancer, currently the number-one cancer killer of women.

As for alcohol, a 1993 NIH study found that two alcoholic drinks per day could raise your estrogen levels enough to increase your risk of breast cancer by 40–100 per cent over women who do not drink at all. In this study, 34 women had their blood levels checked mid-cycle, and were found to have a 31.9 per cent increase in estrogen over women who were not drinking. Of course, it's also been shown that between 1–2 glasses of wine per day for men and 1–3 alcoholic beverages *per week* for women may lower the risk of heart disease. The alcohol raises your "good" cholesterol (HDL), thus reducing the deposits of cholesterol in the arterial walls.

As for illegal drugs, such as cocaine, your risks of suffering a drug-related overdose or other health problem should be your main concern.

bras

In his book *Dressed to Kill: The Link Between Breast Cancer and Bras*, medical anthropologist Sydney Ross Singer raises the question of whether bras cause breast cancer. He compared women in five U.S. cities who wore bras to those who didn't, and concluded that women who wore bras had a higher breast cancer risk. Based on interviews with 4,700 women, Singer and his co-author wife claim that bras constrict the lymph system thus preventing it from "draining and flushing out toxins." The buildup of toxins in breast tissue, according to Singer, triggers lumps, bumps, and cancer.

Medical doctors say this hypothesis is pure nonsense, and point out that if this were true, most breast cancers would not occur in the outer upper quadrant of the breasts where the bras restrict the least. According to Singer, wearing a bra 24 hours a day increases a woman's risk 125-fold, but removing it for 2 weeks "cures" fibrocystic breast condition (which, by the way, does not mean breast cancer). Another reason that doctors discount Singer's hypothesis is that there are many women who do not wear bras who still have fibrocystic breast condition. Doctors call Singer's study either "bad science" or "junk science" because he has not eliminated the influence of other significant breast cancer risk factors, such as diet, for example. One doctor wrote to me that "[Singer's] study is just awful. You could use his methods to prove anything you want."

What Singer may have stumbled across is the issue of the breast being held too close to body temperature. Males with undescended testicles, for example, have a higher incidence of testicular cancer. Scientific literature notes that women who wear tight bras can develop *hyperprolactinemia*, a condition where there's too much prolactin, the hormone that controls milk production, in your system.

Singer also raises the notion that braless cultures seen in Africa or Asia have low rates of breast cancer, while African- and Asian-American women, who do wear bras, have high rates of breast cancer. However, keep in mind that the diet in African and Asian cultures are lower-fat and often high in fish sea vegetables (seaweed), the women have more children, first children *earlier*, and breast-feed longer. In addition, North America is more industrialized. And we know that where there's industry, there's a higher rate of breast cancer anyway, due, possibly, to some differences such as fewer children, later first children, less breast-feeding, and higher longevity rates. So don't burn your bra again just yet, but you can certainly go braless if you like.

Massaging your breasts daily apparently helps get the blood flowing properly. In fact, some theories hold that nipple stimulation may reduce breast cancer risk by clearing free radicals and/or raising the hormone oxytocin and lowering prolactin in the body.

demographics

Who gets breast cancer largely depends on where people live. Industrialized countries have much higher breast cancer rates than underdeveloped countries. Region dramatically affects the rates of breast cancer, but we don't know why. For instance, the breast cancer rate in Switzerland is double that of Spain's—even though they are not that far apart geographically. In California, the rate is double that of Newfoundland's, proving that breast cancer, in North America, can vary from coast to coast.

More interesting, a 1992 *New England Journal of Medicine* article concluded that people migrating from regions with low rates of breast cancer increased their own risk when they entered a country with higher incidences of the disease. This supports the theory that breast cancer is largely due to environmental factors, such as lifestyle, culture, diet, water, and air quality.

The risk of breast cancer in North America is also about 30 per cent higher in urban communities than rural ones, and as a result, is higher in black communities than white. But the incidence is highest in North America, where a woman's lifetime risk of breast cancer is 1 in 8.

The bottom line is that where there's heavy industry, there are higher cancer rates of all kinds. In the United States, the northeastern states comprise the five highest cancer death rates in the U.S., while the rural western and southern states comprise the five lowest cancer death rates. In Canada, British Columbia, Ontario, and Quebec have higher cancer rates than other parts of Canada. In Europe, there are dramatic extremes in cancer death rates: England has the highest cancer mortality rates in the world, while southern Italy has exceptionally low cancer mortality rates.

environmental factors

Environmental factors are extremely important when assessing your risk of breast cancer. While radiation exposure from modern-day X-rays is not a concern, high-dose radiation exposure is. For example, if your breasts were exposed to high-dose radiation, this can increase your risk of breast cancer, especially if you were exposed around the time of your first menstrual period. This could mean either direct radiation from a high-dose X-ray, or from radiation emitted during a nuclear explosion or accident.

Women who live near areas with high levels of radioactive fallout have higher incidences of a variety of cancers, including breast cancer. We know this because women survivors of Hiroshima and Nagasaki were extensively followed. The breast cancer rates dramatically rose within the entire female population, but particularly rose within younger women in their teens and 20s. The most recent conclusion of this data is that the highest number of breast cancer cases was seen in women who were less than 10 years old when they were exposed to fallout. Women who were older when exposed did not seem to be vulnerable to this effect. It is possible that breasts become more resistant to radiation as they mature.

Similar studies have backed up this early radiation exposure risk. In North America, women who were checked for tuberculosis as children using fluoroscopy (high-dose X-rays where the picture was taken as the child inhaled) in the 1930s and 1940s were found to have higher rates of breast cancer. Moreover, a Rochester study showed that women treated with radiation for mastitis (bacterial breast infection) from the 1920s to the 1960s also had higher rates of breast cancer. The same goes for women treated with radiation as children for acne, enlarged thymus glands (used in infants), and anyone subjected to the equivalent of one X-ray per week for two years in childhood, as in people with scoliosis (abnormal curvature of the spine), for example.

Some studies have found that the increase in risk is directly proportional to the radiation dose. During the 1930s and 1940s, radiation was also widely used to determine fetal positions in prenatal care (pelvimetry, which exposed the fetal breast tissue to radiation), and was also used to treat asthma, pneumonia, whooping cough, and even hyperthyroidism (today, radioactive iodine is used, which is not linked to breast cancer). Let's not forget the radiation used to treat congenital heart problems, as well as those standard TB exams most employers demanded between 1920 and 1960. Radiation was also widely used by chiropractors to determine spinal column alignment, and shoe retailers, who used high-dose X-rays on the feet to determine a person's shoe size.

In his book *Preventing Breast Cancer: The Story of a Major, Proven, Preventable Cause of This Disease* (1995), John W. Gofman concludes that about 75 per cent of breast cancer cases are largely due to past medical-related radiation. In other words, according to Gofman, women who received radiation as children or young women may be able to link their breast cancers to that period in their life. He also suggests that much of the radiation therapy between the 1920s and 1960s was probably poorly documented; that is, much more radiation therapy was done than we think. Gofman states that 75 per cent of the women who have recently had breast cancer or are currently diagnosed would probably never have developed it if medicine had never used irradiation. Gofman also states that there is no safe level of radiation; even low-dose radiation can cause cancer, but at much lower rates than high-dose radiation.

electromagnetic fields

Researchers are still trying to see if electromagnetic fields—areas near power lines—can predispose people who live near them or people who work under them, to higher rates of cancer. Some studies have found the increase in breast cancer risk is directly proportional to the radiation dose.

environmental estrogens

The role of chemical pollutants seems to be far more ominous than any single environmental factor. In 1994, a major discovery led many medical researchers and environmental scientists to the same conclusion: life on planet Earth is being threatened by a group of substances known as environmental estrogens. A very long grocery list of organic chemicals, found in various pesticides and plastics, are transforming in the natural environment into a substance that is identical to the female hormone estrogen. And the results are absolutely disastrous, threatening not only human fertility, but contributing to an epidemic of reproductive cancers, such as breast cancer in women and testicular cancer in men. These chemicals are also disrupting several wildlife species, who are now being born as hermaphrodites or sterile. In Florida, for example, the majority of male alligators are sterile as a result of either non-developed or abnormally shaped penises. A chemical spill in nearby waters was found to be the culprit, which was having an estrogenic effect on the alligators' natural habitat.

One of the worst organic chemical culprits is nonylphenol, a substance which is used in hundreds of everyday consumer products: detergents, toiletries, cosmetics, and oils. It also lines the insides of canned goods; it's found in various plastic food wraps; it's found in spermicides and contraceptive foam, and a variety of other products. The scientific literature is slowly becoming saturated with findings linking one organic chemical after another to reproductive cancers and endocrine disruption in both wildlife and humans.

Organic chemicals are in the air we breathe from numerous air pollutants; the food preservatives used in numerous canned and packaged goods; and in the pesticides used on fresh produce. These chemicals then contaminate the water and soil, which contaminate the entire human food chain. Some suggest that environmental estrogens are "feminizing" the planet. Some suggest that women are perhaps being overloaded with estrogen, which may be associated with the rise of estrogen-dependent cancers, as well as estrogen-related conditions, such as endometriosis and fibroids.

Estrogen pollutants are also thought to accumulate in fatty tissues (estrogen pollutants are fat). Since women generally carry more body fat than men, women may be accumulating more of these toxins. Some studies have already found that women with breast cancer tended to have higher concentrations of the organochlorines (a type of manufactured chemical) DDT, DDE, or PCBs in their fat tissue. In fact, elevated levels of DDE in the blood have been directly linked to a fourfold increase of breast cancer in the United States. We already know that dioxins, also organocholorines, are associated with endometriosis. It's estimated that billions of gallons of organochlorines have been released onto an unsuspecting environment. Since these chemicals are resistant to breaking down, they're spread around the world through the air and water, exposing us to toxins in our food, groundwater, surface water, and air. According to a 1992 Greenpeace report on chlorine and human health, no industrial organochlorines are known to be *non*-toxic.

Pesticides are major contributors to the environmental estrogen problem, one of the most notorious of which is DDT. DDT stands for dichloro-diphenyl-trichlore-ethane and was banned in most industrialized countries by the mid-1970s. But even though DDT has been pretty much banned in most countries since 1972, it remains active in the environment for 25 to 30 years.

There is some promising news, however. Health Canada found that DDT levels in breast milk dropped from roughly 150 parts per billion (ppb) in 1967 to less than 15 ppb in 1986, and that they are still falling. PCBs (polychlorinated biphenyl), which are also banned in North America, fell from 30 ppb to about 5 in Canada, while in the United States, the Environmental Protection Agency (EPA) reports that PCB levels in Lake Michigan trout dropped from 23 parts per million (ppm) in 1974 to 3 ppm in 1993, still above the 2 ppm safety limit, though.

Israel Bans Toxic Substances

One of the strongest cases to link pesticides such as DDT to breast cancer is the Israeli pesticide ban of the 1970s. Faced with one of the highest breast cancer rates in the world by the 1970s, the Israeli government decided to ban three pesticides: a-BHC (benzine hexachloride, or hexachlorocyclohexane), y-BHC (lindane), and DDT. Israel's agricultural boom in the 1960s and 1970s had led to the presence of far higher concentrations of these pesticides than in countries like the United States. For example, concentrations of DDE, the DDT by-product, were about 500 per cent higher in Israeli milk than U.S. milk prior to the ban. It was reported that the breast cancer mortality rate was double that of countries with similar fat consumption. So, it was decided that these three pesticides were to be phased out by 1978. Between 1976 and 1986 Israel's breast cancer rate was reported to have dropped by nearly 8 per cent, even though breast cancer rates were rising everywhere else. Factor in the global increase of breast cancer rates at the time, and the statistic you get is a 20 per cent drop.

A 1990 paper published in the *Annals of the New York Academy of Science* concluded that the drop in breast cancer rates in Israel were directly linked to the country's ban on pesticides.

Israeli statistics criticized

Not everyone buys the Israeli breast cancer story, however. Many critics point out that there were simply too many other factors not taken into consideration. For example, between 1976 and 1986, were more women having children? Were more women having children earlier? Was there an increase in breast-feeding? And what about immigration from other countries with lower breast cancer rates?

One critic argues that the study that reported the drop in breast cancer rates was flawed in that it did not account for year-to-year natural fluctuations in cancer rates. He argues that had the study compared breast cancer rates for the years 1975 and 1985, instead of 1976 and 1986, it would have found a 62 per cent increase in breast cancer deaths in young women. And, had the study looked at mortality data from 1965 to 1988, it would have found that the rate of breast cancer in Israel remained almost constant.

estrogen

High levels of estrogen seem to be markers for increased risk of breast cancer. The estrogen question is complicated, however, since there are times in your life when estrogen levels are high, such as during pregnancy or during certain times in your menstrual cycle. Fat cells also make estrogen, but this isn't a concern until after menopause (see chapter 1). Sources of extra estrogen include:

- Exposure to DES (diethylstilbestrol), a drug administered to pregnant women from the 1940s to the 1970s to prevent miscarriage. DES daughters are at risk for a variety of reproductive cancers, mainly vaginal and cervical. Breast cancer is more likely if you are a DES daughter, however. For more information, contact the DES Cancer Network at 510-465-4011.
- Hormone replacement therapy (see chapter 1) or birth control pills after age 35.
- Dietary fat. This is not an external source of estrogen, but may contribute to your fat cells' production of estrogen if the fat you eat makes you fat! (See What to Eat at the end of this chapter.)
- Hormone-fed produce. (See What To Eat.)
- Environmental estrogens. (See pages 93–96.)

Please keep in mind, though, that estrogen levels are hard to calculate and are often misread by various researchers. The level can vary with the time of day, menstrual cycle, pregnancy, and lactation. Studies that base their conclusions on a single measurement of estrogen in women may show confusing or contradictory results. The reading will be true for each woman at the *time* it was taken. However, the degree to which the reading can be taken as an indicator of that woman's overall estrogen exposure is questionable.

exercise

Like diet, exercise also plays a huge role in lowering our risk of a variety of health problems. Breast cancer is one of those. The more we exercise, the more fat we burn, the more oxygen is carried to our muscles, and the better our bodies work.

On average, women who do four hours of exercise a week may reduce their risks of premenopausal breast cancer by as much as 58 per cent; women with no children lower their risks by 27 per cent, while women with children lower their risks by as much as 72 per cent. The younger you begin regular exercise, the more you may be protected from breast cancer. Even so, women who don't get started until later in life are still more protected than women who are sedentary.

However, exercise is only *associated* with lower breast cancer risk. We don't know what other factors are at work. Are both diet and exercise and some other unknown factor associated with breast cancer risk? Are women who are predisposed to breast cancer less inclined to exercise anyway? We just don't know. What does happen with strenuous exercise is that ovarian function is decreased and hence estrogen levels are lower. In athletes, for example, periods may stop altogether (called amenorrhea), which does lower breast cancer risk. What we also know is that people who exercise regularly tend to eat better.

According to a number of studies, the best forms of exercise are jogging, racquet sports, swimming, strenuous walking, and weightlifting. It's suggested that a range of activities is the best kind of program (probably because it relieves boredom and monotony). (See "How To Move" at the end of this chapter.)

hormone replacement therapy (HRT)

(For a detailed discussion of HRT see pages 14–25.)

menstrual history

Unfortunately, your menstrual history can apparently affect your risk of breast cancer, but many experts disagree about how significant a role it truly plays in the big picture.

One risk factor is what experts call "early menarche." Menarche refers to your first period; early menarche means that you got your first period prior to age 12. This seemingly trivial detail also means that you've been making estrogen longer than the average woman, which is the reason that this is even looked at.

Menarche levels can vary enormously. The average age of menarche is 12.8 in the United States and 17 in China. Some researchers say this is why breast cancer occurrence in China is a third that of the U.S. And even within China, provinces with later menarche tend to have lower rates of breast cancer.

Another risk factor is menstrual cycle length. If your cycles are either longer (less evidence for this) or shorter (more evidence for this) than average (an average cycle is anywhere from 26–29 days), your breast cancer risk increases by as high as 50 per cent. It's believed that shorter or longer cycles indicate a hormonal imbalance, which *may* contribute to an increased breast cancer risk. Shorter cycles also indicate that you're making more estrogen than women with longer cycles.

pregnancy history

Your pregnancy history is a huge factor in determining your overall risk of breast cancer. In fact, according to a 1751 edition of the *Chambers Encyclopedia*, breast cancer is described as "a most dread disease, particularly of the celibate and barren." To a large extent, this is still true today. For example, according to the National Cancer Institute (NCI), lesbians are two to three times more likely to develop breast cancer than heterosexual women, while child-free women are 50 per cent more likely to develop breast cancer than women who gave birth to children before age 35. Curiously, if you bear your first child after 35, your pregnancy no longer offers you the same protection against breast cancer—*unless you decide to breast-feed.*

abortion

Your pregnancy history can be a paradox in terms of breast cancer risk. For example, the more full-term pregnancies a women has, the lower her risk of developing breast cancer after menopause. However, women who've had children may be more likely to get breast cancer before they are 35. Also, if the pregnancy was interrupted through a therapeutic abortion (surgical termination of a pregnancy as opposed to a miscarriage), some studies indicate that the risks of breast cancer may increase. Here's why:

Once you become pregnant, even if the pregnancy is terminated, your breasts have changed in structure. The hormonal symphony that controls the pregnancy causes cellular changes in your breasts as well as tissue growth. Throughout the pregnancy, the breasts continue to change until they reach their final maturation prior to delivery, when you're physically able to breast-feed. However, if a pregnancy ends in the first trimester, all the changes your breasts have been going through suddenly stop, making the cells less stable and possibly more vulnerable to cancer.

Even if subsequent pregnancies go to term, your risks are apparently slightly increased as a result of an abortion. Some studies argue that the more abortions you have, the greater your risk, but this is highly debatable. Studies remain inconclusive here. In women who carry their first baby to term the risk of breast cancer is reduced by roughly 50 per cent. So, what we can say at this point is that women who abort may be at greater risk if they're 18 or under, they're aborting after 8 weeks, or breast cancer runs in their family. Interestingly, one study found that women who aborted, but later breast-fed, did not seem to have an increased risk of breast cancer.

weight

The more fat your culture eats, the higher the rate of breast cancer in your cultural group. This may be due to the fat eaten, or to other dietary or lifestyle differences between cultures. However, the more fat on your body, the greater your risk of breast cancer. That's because fat cells store estrogen and manufacture it, increasing your risk of estrogen-dependent cancers, as well as a number of other diseases.

apples and pears

While we can all do something about our weight, it's difficult to do much about our body shapes. Unfortunately, one study has actually linked body shapes to breast cancer risk. According to the study, pear-shaped figures, where more weight is carried around the hips and thighs, are less at risk for breast cancer than apple-shaped figures, where more weight is carried around the waist than the hips and thighs.

Lots of data indicates that the fat in our spare-tire area is more metabolically active than the fat on our thighs, hips, and rear ends. The "apple-shape" theory was refuted by researchers from the Memorial Sloan-Kettering Cancer Center, who reported in 1993 that they found no such link.

Interestingly, smoking changes fat metabolism so that the fat is distributed more in the spare-tire area; however, this may not increase your risk of breast cancer, since smoking is also linked to earlier menopause.

Should You Be Worried?

Most women grossly overestimate their risk of breast cancer by as much as four times. If you're worried about it, however, it's probably worth it it seek counselling, for some peace of mind, and a more realistic perspective. If you're looking for answers solely based on "known" risk factors, you probably won't get much more than you would from a tea-leaf reading, because 70 per cent of the women who develop breast cancer do not have any of the known risk factors. In the meantime, use the following guidelines to help you make your decision about counselling:

You have reason to worry about breast cancer over the age of 50 if:

1. You have a first-degree relative (mother, sister, or daughter) who has a history of breast cancer.
2. You have a first-degree relative (mother, sister, or daughter) who has a history of colon, ovarian, or endometrial cancer.
3. You yourself had breast cancer, colon, ovarian, or endometrial cancer.
4. Other than mammography and diagnostic chest X-rays, you've been exposed to high-dose X-rays or high-dose radiation to your chest area. (Fluoroscopy or nuclear fallout.)
5. You have dense breast tissue (more problems with interpreting mammogram results).
6. You have had breast biopsies done for benign breast problems, excluding fibroadenomas (benign breast tumours).
7. You had an early menarche (early period).
8. You did not breast-feed (minor).
9. You are obese or eat large amounts of fat (minor).
10. You have never been pregnant (minor).
11. You are a DES daughter (minor).

You MAY have reason to worry about breast cancer under or over the age of 50 if:

1. You have high estrogen levels (shown on a blood test).
2. You have more years of education than average (there are some cultural/lifestyle risks associated with this).
3. You don't eat many fruits or vegetables.
4. You live in a highly industrialized area with a lot of chemical plants nearby.
5. You're exposed to estrogenic chemicals in your work or residence.

genetic screening

Many cancers run in families, but it's particularly true with breast, ovarian, and colon cancers. That's why research into finding specific cancer genes is an important step in identifying women at risk.

"First-degree" relatives—parents, siblings, and children—determine whether you have a strong family history of breast cancer. That means that in order to qualify, either your mother or sister, and on rare occasions, your daughter, would have been diagnosed with breast cancer. The younger they were at the time of their diagnosis, the more at risk you are. Grandmothers, great-aunts, and paternal relatives are not as crucial in determining family histories. However, if breast cancer was diagnosed in your maternal aunt (your mother's sister), there is a stronger likelihood that the disease runs in the family. Familial breast cancer, however, accounts for only 5–10 per cent of all breast cancers diagnosed. One study also found that daughters of men with prostate cancer were at a higher risk of developing breast cancer.

what about genes?

Since about 1940, researchers have known that cancer is caused by mutating cells. This process used to be attributed to aging cells in aging bodies, but we now know that there are genes that *control* mutation. And some genes have more control over mutation than others.

Oncogenes are genes that can transform a cell into a tumour cell. These are dormant genes that absorb various external "hits" until they switch on and tell our cells to mutate. Some of us will never turn on our oncogenes, but many of us will. So the question is, are there specific genes that make us more susceptible to a carcinogen, such as tobacco or pesticides, for example.

As for specific cancer genes that are present in the sperm and egg when we reproduce, only a small number of cancers have so far been shown to be genetically inherited in this way. Most research is trying to pin down what switches on some oncogenes and not others.

the breast cancer gene

Several inherited abnormal genes can cause susceptibility to certain cancers, including the genes BRCA1, BRCA2, BRCA3, hMLH1 and hMLH2. The most well known breast cancer gene that has been isolated is BRCA1, and women who have this gene are more susceptible to breast cancer than those who don't. The BRCA1 is a dominant gene, but in our bodies behaves like a recessive gene. It kicks into action when its normal partner gene (which may be a tumour suppresser gene) is either lost or becomes inactive.

It's possible to be screened for BRCA1, but doing mass screenings is not very useful because this gene accounts for only 4–5 per cent of all breast cancers. It is also found in women who don't get breast cancer and who come from low-risk families. And since we don't know what finding BRCA1 in a woman without a high-risk family means, screening everyone would wind up scaring people for no good reason. In addition, there are probably many other genes—good and bad—that play a role in the development of breast cancer; we just haven't found all of them yet.

Another problem with screening is that there is no way to tell a woman without the BRCA1 gene that she's *not* at risk for breast cancer since there are so many other factors involved. At this point, the reasoning is that it's better to spend this money on something that we know for a fact can save lives.

It's estimated that 1 in 300 women carry this gene and that it's responsible for 4 per cent of all breast cancer cases. In younger women, however, the BRCA1 gene is implicated in 25 per cent of cases. If you are BRCA1-positive, it's estimated, using data from high-risk families, that there is an 85 per cent chance of developing breast cancer before age 80, although about 50 per cent of women who fall into this group will develop the disease before they are 50. It's also been found that women who are BRCA1-positive come from families in which half of all female members are affected. If you are BRCA1-positive and come from a low-risk family, nobody knows for sure what this means, if indeed it means anything at all.

about genetic testing

In order to determine whether the cancer in your family is genetic, it's recommended that you and your family go for genetic counselling. The genetic counsellor will document your family history to check if you say yes to any of the following statements:

1. Cancers occur in three or more family members.
2. Cancers in your family occur before age 40.
3. A person in your family developed more than one cancer; for example, separate cancers in each breast; or ovarian and breast cancer.

4. Family members have "closely related" cancers; for example, breast, ovarian, colon, endometrial, and uterine (these are all hormone-related).

The implications of a positive or negative result need to be considered carefully. Again, neither result is a guarantee of cancer or no cancer in your lifetime. If necessary, a genetic counsellor will recommend screening methods such as screening mammogram or colonoscopy. Some experts recommend that mammograms begin at age 25 if you're considered at high risk for breast cancer, and age 20 if your family members develop breast cancer in their 30s. Not all experts agree with these recommendations, however.

More controversy surrounds other recommendations to women with a high-risk family who have the BRCA1 gene. Recommendations may involve a bilateral mastectomy (removal of both breasts), oophorectomy (removal of the ovaries), and the drug tamoxifen as prevention therapy (see pages 113–116). The pros and cons of each of these recommendations must be thoroughly discussed with more than one cancer expert.

ethics of breast cancer gene testing

Imagine a subway platform. The northbound platform is crowded; in fact, jammed with people. The southbound platform is practically empty, with just a few people comfortably sitting down on the benches provided. Due to mechanical problems, only one train is available. You have the power, however, to decide which platform to send the train. Do you choose the crowded or sparse platform? A reasonable person might choose to send the train to the crowded platform because, presumably, more people would benefit. Yet a situation exists in breast cancer research right now, where the train has been sent to the sparse platform. The majority of breast cancer research is devoted to roughly 5 per cent of the overall breast cancer population, ignoring the needs of the majority. Why is that? And can we continue to refuse "train service" to the crowded platform? In other words, is it fair that almost all resources should be directed toward genetic causes of breast cancer instead of looking at other ways to prevent this disease?

In the 1970s, 1980s, and early 1990s, mammography screening, although the centre of fierce debate, was a funding magnet. In the wake of the still-unresolved mammography screening guidelines (see pages 108–110), a new screening debate, fraught with similar but deeper ethical issues, has emerged: genetic screening.

reopening old wounds

The financial and emotional toll of breast cancer gene screening is in some ways analogous to the issues raised over mammography screening in 1976, when researchers criticized the motives and methods behind it. The issue at that time was whether the money spent on mammography could be better spent in other areas of cancer prevention and treatment. Then there were the hidden costs: since mammograms were inaccurate, a large number of women would need to undergo investigative surgery, general anesthesia, and ultimately pay the bill. Other socioeconomic costs not raised at the time had to do with absenteeism and lost productivity. In 1988 the emotional costs of mammography in younger women (under age 50) resulting from both false-positive and false-negative results was also brought up. There are uncomfortable similarities between the concerns raised in 1988 over the emotional toll of inaccurate mammography results and the uncertainty over what genetic testing results really "predict."

the downside of genetic testing

Testing for genetic mutations in presymptomatic women who come from high-risk families is producing a registry of confidential information that can perhaps be more damaging to the future of the affected woman or families than the genetic mutation itself. Some of the following represent dilemmas regarding testing for the breast cancer gene:

1. *Who owns this information?* It is currently unclear whether a woman who tests positive for a breast cancer gene mutation can keep the information confidential.
2. *How will this information be used?* The film *Gattica* dramatizes the results of a genetically obsessed culture. In this film, one's genetic makeup determines one's eligibility for education, employment, and social status, even though the film's protagonist makes it clear that "genoism" (a word in the film that meant discrimination against people with genetic "defects" or mutations) is against the law. *Gattica* shows us a world that is not as futuristic as we might hope; a world where every strand of hair or eyelash serves as one's genetic resumé.

   Insurance companies in the U.S. already practice a form of "genoism" with clauses that prevent people with "pre-existing conditions" from receiving health care insurance. Could insurers in the near future require, for example, BRCA-positive women to undergo a bilateral prophylactic mastectomy as a condition of coverage? Or would health insurance premiums simply become unaffordable for BRCA-positive women, or the families of positive women? As for denying employment to BRCA-positive women, while the Equal Employment Opportunity Commission (EEOC) considers genetic discrimination unethical under the 1990 American with Disabilities Act (ADA), its powers are limited. Given this, what would stop employers from requiring that BRCA-positive women undergo a bilateral prophylactic mastectomy as a condition of hiring?

3. *BRCA Daughters*. First, at what point does a mother tell her daughter that she is BRCA-positive? At 21? At 16? At birth? While there are guidelines in place that prohibit genetic testing in girls under 18, there is no way to enforce that a BRCA-positive woman withhold her *own* testing results from her daughter. The emotional impact of a daughter knowing that she carries a "defect" may be an unfair burden. How will this information affect other decisions this daughter makes, ranging from career choices to contraception methods, to child-bearing?

   Second, would BRCA screening become available prenatally? Would BRCA-positive pregnancies be terminated? In India, for example, little girls are aborted because they are viewed as economic burdens on families; in kind, little girls who grow up to be breast cancer patients may be viewed as economic burdens.

is getting tested harmful?

Genetic testing can be harmful, depending on how you're interpreting the news, or who is interpreting it for you. If you have inadequate genetic counselling (which happens a lot!), critics of genetic testing state that misunderstood genetic information can do enormous damage.

It's important to consider the following before deciding to get tested:

Testing Negative. Testing negative is never a true negative since the test is not an accurate prediction of one's future health. Some women mistakenly interpret a negative result to mean that they will never develop any form of breast cancer. If other women in your family are being tested at the same time, the women in the family who test negative may suffer from "survivor's guilt," if other women test positive.

Testing Positive. On the flip side, testing positive is not necessarily a guarantee of breast cancer, although there is certainly a greater likelihood of a BRCA-positive woman developing breast cancer. The issue of harm should be examined in the context of whether a still-healthy, presymptomatic woman should sacrifice her emotional health. Women who test positive are more likely to suffer from anxiety, depression, and hopelessness, strained relationships with family members, and even employment and insurance discrimination. A more frightening scenario is suicide, which has been linked, for example, to positive mammograms.

Harmful interventions. Right now, women who test positive for a breast cancer gene are recommended for more intensive mammography screening at very early ages of 20 or 25. In light of the question of damage from mammography (see page 110), this may, in fact, be putting women at greater risk for breast cancer. More controversy surrounds the questionable prophylactic therapies available to women (see page 116) as well as the tamoxifen controversy (see pages 113–116). All of these prophylactic therapies ask women to sacrifice their health before they show symptoms of a disease.

Ageism. The trend to screen younger populations for breast cancer yet refuse "train service" to the crowded platform populated by older women at risk for breast cancer not only demonstrates that there is a greater value placed on the lives of younger women than older women, but asks the majority of breast cancer victims to sacrifice their health.

Rich versus Poor. Justice demands that women should be eligible for testing regardless of ethnic background, ability to pay, and so forth. History teaches us different lessons about justice and breast cancer. In the U.S., poor women have lower survival rates of breast cancer than affluent women because they have less access to screening and health care delivery.

So once out of the research setting and into the service sector, genetic screening may widen the gap between the rich and poor, allowing the rich more options with respect to screening. And even if genetic screening continues to be accessible through research trials, that would mean poor women are forced into becoming research subjects if they want to be tested. Currently, mammography screening in the U.S. targets women who can afford it. Will genetic testing follow a similar marketing plan?

Vulnerable populations. Finally, is breast cancer gene testing an uncontrolled experiment on a vulnerable population? Because of past medical abuses involving women's reproductive organs, the public has demanded stronger regulations to protect them, labelling those with reproductive potential "vulnerable," thus banning them from medical research. Testing premenopausal women for the breast cancer gene has implications for their reproductive organs: positive women may be recommended for prophylactic treatments that have questionable benefits. Unless the risks of certain procedures or treatments are well established, and women are informed of all the potential risks, women's reproductive organs are in danger of being abused once again.

established benefits of genetic research

Breast cancer gene researchers maintain that continuing to map specific genes linked to breast cancer could, one day, lead to a cure for breast cancer. If the mutated gene responsible for breast cancer, and other cancers, could be manipulated somehow prior to being "switched on," we'd have a cure for breast cancer. As for the issue of serving the needs of the few while ignoring the needs of the many, researchers maintain that BRCA1, 2, and 3 represent the genes they've found to date. By continuing to fund more genetic research, we may be able to find genes that are relevant in the majority of breast cancers. While this certainly is an intriguing notion, does it justify screening women for breast cancer genes today when there is no way to manipulate the gene currently? Possibly.

There are potential benefits in store for both BRCA-positive and -negative women. Women who test negative may experience less anxiety about their risk. And women who test positive may benefit from planning a more rigorous detection strategy so that they may find cancer earlier and increase their chances of survival. Moreover, they may opt for prophylactic therapies which, although questionable, are still potentially life-saving measures. Moreover, some women benefit from knowing the "bad news" earlier.

more harm than good?

All of the potential benefits of genetic screening can only be delivered in the presence of good counselling, not *simply* counselling. In the same way that mammography demands a good pathologist on the scene to interpret the mammogram, genetic testing demands proper counselling before and after testing. Without proper counselling, critics of testing compare handing out test results to handing a loaded gun to a child. But that is not their worst fear. *There are not enough counsellors to go around.* In the U.S., for example, roughly 12 million people could benefit from genetic counselling, but there are only 1,000 trained genetic counsellors, 40 of whom actually work in clinical cancer centres.

That said, even in the presence of good, even great, counselling, the options are still lousy. There is currently no proven prophylactic therapy for breast cancer. Giving tamoxifen to presymptomatic women has been questioned by critics on ethical grounds. Meanwhile, chopping off a woman's healthy breasts is a questionable practice; and exposing under-40 breasts to frequent mammograms may also expose them to harmful radiation.

And is it ethical to predict one possible future, without any sound preventive therapy? In other words, what is the purpose of doing "preventive screening" unless a therapy exists that can clearly prevent the disease?

profiting from frightened women?

Some genetic counsellors and health writers believe that the fear over breast cancer risk is good for business. In other words, there are financial incentives for some companies to sell genetic tests. Clearly, genetic testing is a more profitable venture than lifestyle counselling. Nobody makes money if a woman at risk for breast cancer cuts out red meat; lots of people make money when she decides to go for genetic testing, bringing along four sisters, two aunts, and a grandmother.

With all of the unanswered ethical questions breast cancer gene testing raises for women and society in general, coupled with the notion that it serves fewer than 10 per cent of women with breast cancer, allocating most of our resources to genetic research and testing seems at best, unjust.

mammography guidelines at 50

Depending on what you read and what expert you talk to, you will probably hear two sets of mammography screening guidelines: "mammography at 50" and "mammography at 40." The good news is that now that you're turning 50, the guidelines are a lot clearer. That's because no one disagrees with the benefits of routine breast screening at 50.

Advocates of screening at 50 point out that breast cancer incidence per 100,000 women rises after age 50, that is, after menopause, which is why screening should begin at this time. The truth is, the rate of increased risk is actually highest *until* age 50, when the rate of increase drops slightly.

Another theory is that denser breast tissue, which is premenopausal breast tissue, and hence, younger than 50, is more difficult to compress and therefore more difficult to read and interpret. As for dense breast tissue, the younger the woman, the less fatty the breast tissue, and hence, the harder it is to read and interpret the mammogram. The older the woman, the fattier the breast tissue, and hence the easier it is to read and interpret the mammogram.

Only one-fifth of all abnormalities found on mammograms turns out to be malignant. In the U.S., out of the roughly 600,000 breast biopsies done annually for mammographic abnormalities, only 20–30 per cent at best are actually malignant. Therefore, 580,000 women will go through the emotional roller coaster associated with breast biopsies. In fact, the emotional toll of being told the mammogram is positive has actually been costed out in dollars and cents; it is not an insignificant amount.

who recommends what?

The American Cancer Society recommends that women 40 or older have annual mammograms, while the National Cancer Institute recommends that women 40 or older have mammograms every one or two years. If you haven't gone yet, don't worry about it, because...

The American College of Obstetricians and Gynecologists, the American College of Radiologists and their Canadian, British, Swedish, Dutch, and Italian counterparts recommend mammographies annually for women 50 or older; the American College of Physicians recommends mammograms every two years for women 50 or older. In this age group, routine mammography every 2–3 years seems to reduce annual breast cancer mortality rates by 20–40 per cent.

The American Medical Association, the National Cancer Institute, and the American Cancer Society *were* recommending screenings every one or two years for women 40 or older; in light of a 1992 Canadian study (which many experts dismissed as flawed), guidelines went into flux, and seem to be reverting to screening at 50 anyway.

what should you do?

You have to make your breast cancer screening decision based on your level of personal comfort. Whether you go every year, or once every two years, or not at all, it's important to check your breasts monthly for lumps (see pages 121–122). If you are anxious because you think you should have been screened earlier but weren't, take comfort in the fact that the science on this is inconclusive. Since your breasts radically change after menopause in terms of denseness, having what the American Medical Association recommends as a baseline mammogram sometime between 35–39 which, in theory, can be compared to future mammograms, is probably not very useful.

Here are some other guidelines to use in making your screening decision: If you find a suspicious lump, your doctor may recommend mammography to help determine what's going on. No matter how old you are, or what your risk factors are, have it. Period. If there's a question as to your screening centre's credibility, from word of mouth, for example, or a bad experience, get a second mammogram done at another centre.

If you have a family history of estrogen-dependent cancers, such as breast, ovarian, or colon cancers, earlier routine screening at age 40 may be a good idea, and can offer you some comfort. Many experts recommend that with this kind of history, annual screening after age 40 is a good idea. If your mother, sister, or grandmother had breast cancer, you may even want to consider mammography at 35. For the rest of the population, lifestyle and dietary adjustments is the recipe for prevention. Then, routine screening started at the guideline age you're comfortable with makes the most sense.

Regardless of your age, do breast self-exam (BSE) and familiarize yourself with your breasts so you'll be equipped to notice anything unusual. You should also make sure that a manual breast exam is performed by your doctor each year when you go for your Pap smear.

maximizing mammography

Outside of feeling your own breasts regularly, you have to make the best of mammography, which currently carries between a 10–15 per cent false-negative rate and a much higher false-positive rate.

Many women avoid even routine mammography beyond age 50 because they fear pain, radiation, or the possibility of a positive result. Other barriers to mammography include a lack of education about when and why to have one, the lack of transportation to a screening centre, language difficulties, cultural issues, and even illiteracy. Clearly, it's impossible for all of these barriers to be removed, but if you have a relative or friend, for example, who refuses to have a mammogram because of some of these barriers, you can help to educate her by translating or explaining information you, yourself, receive, or by accompanying her to a physician who can help explain screening to her.

Getting the Most Out of Your Mammogram

Mammography standards vary from screening centre to screening centre. To get the most out of your mammogram, consider the following:

1. Go to a reliable screening centre, one that specializes in mammograms, and does at least 20–30 mammograms each day.
2. The image of the breast on the X-ray must be of the highest quality. Good equipment used only for mammography, and purchased no later than three years ago, is your best bet. Cheap or older equipment used by a cut-rate centre will be of no value to you, and could deliver false positives. Ask about the age of your clinic's equipment.
3. A dedicated, experienced technician specially trained in mammography must perform the screening, while, ideally, you should ask if the radiologist interpreting your mammogram specializes in breast radiology. This is not as common as it is slowly becoming. Now some specialists recommend that at least two experienced radiologists read and interpret mammogram results. This is expensive. And if you have two radiologists who do not specialize in reading mammography, you're probably no further ahead. So, ask at your mammogram facility: how many mammograms has the radiologist read?; what is the facility's call-back record?; that is, how many second looks does the facility do? A reasonable number is about 10 per cent or less. A high call-back rate is suspicious because it suggests that the radiologist may be insecure about the readings and keeps rechecking for tiny little things. If the facility doesn't know the call-back record, go elsewhere; it's a sign that there isn't very good quality control there.
4. For the mammogram to be as accurate as possible, there must be maximum compression on the breast, so the procedure may hurt a little bit. Compression also reduces the amount of radiation required. Experts suggest going for your mammogram after your period, when your breasts are least tender. You can also take an over-the-counter painkiller an hour before the test.
5. Ask how much time per patient is spent in the mammography room. Anything less than 20 minutes per patient is too fast!
6. A physical examination of the breasts by a trained nurse or qualified physician *must* accompany the mammogram. Before you go, however, you may want to see your doctor first, who will document any concerns on your mammogram requisition. In fact, the best screening facilities have the radiologist do the clinical exam, read the mammogram, and perform an ultrasound. That way, when it comes time to interpret the mammogram, the radiologist has all the information components needed to interpret it as accurately as possible.
7. Don't wear any talcum powder, deodorant, or lotions on your upper body the day you're scheduled. Little flecks can get on the plates and interfere with the results.

interpreting results

Ten radiologists can have 10 interpretations of a mammogram, and 10 different recommendations in terms of what next. Variations in mammogram interpretations have to do with several areas:

- *Visual observations*. Some radiologists observe a lesion in a given film, while another may miss it altogether.
- *Perception*. One tumour (a.k.a. "mass") may be perceived as "probably benign" by radiologist A and "probably cancerous" by radiologist B. It depends on the radiologist's personality and perspective.
- *Concern*. Some radiologists follow up every abnormality observed, no matter how small, with further tests, while others reserve follow-up tests for only "highly suspicious" abnormalities. Again, it depends on the personality of the radiologist looking at the film.
- *Variables*. Your age, size of breasts, medical history, and quality of mammography equipment also affect interpretation.

Studies show that mammogram interpretations vary so much, many radiologists failed to identify some patients with cancer. In fact, almost 30 per cent of the cancers in one study were incorrectly categorized when the films were originally interpreted in 1987.

Many experts recommend that since radiologists differ in what they catch or miss, using two observers for one mammogram may be the best route, but other experts point out that one mammographer solely specializing in breast radiology may still be better than two who do not specialize in this area. For what it's worth, in Sweden, where mammography interpretation and standards are considered the best in the world, two radiologists per mammogram has increased the cancer detection rate by 15 per cent.

prevention strategies for breast cancer

If you're considered at "high risk" for breast cancer (and as mentioned earlier, this is a meaningless term, as 70 per cent of women who develop breast cancer have no known risk factors), the following are the prevention programs that are on offer. Many experts believe that making some simple lifestyle changes may be better than some of these options. And what's currently being sold to you as prevention may cause more health problems in the long run.

the truth about tamoxifen

Tamoxifen, the very same drug used to treat estrogen-receptor positive breast cancer, was approved by the FDA in 1998 "to reduce the incidence of breast cancer in women at high risk." This is different than approving tamoxifen as a "prevention drug" for breast cancer, especially since there is no proof that tamoxifen can prevent breast cancer.

Here's how tamoxifen got approved as a prevention drug. In 1992, $68 million was allocated to the Breast Cancer Study (incorrectly referred to by the media as the "breast cancer prevention trial"). The Breast Cancer Study was conducted throughout the United States and Canada. It included 13,000 women at high risk for invasive breast cancer. Half of the women took tamoxifen (20 mg/day) and half took a placebo (a dummy pill consisting of sugar and water). The women in the study were at least 35, and had a combination of risks that made their chances of developing breast cancer relatively high. These risk factors comprised women who were over 60; women with a family history of breast cancer; women with an early puberty, and women with a history of suspicious or benign lumps in the breast.

The women were followed for 4.2 years. In the tamoxifen group, 2.2 per cent developed breast cancer, compared to 4.3 per cent in the placebo group. That is why it is reported that tamoxifen can cut the risk of breast cancer "in half." What was not reported, however, is that the numbers of deaths from breast cancer *equalled* the number of deaths from tamoxifen's side effects (endometrial cancer, blood clots, and stroke). In other words, the study revealed that there was a reduction of 2.9 cases of breast cancer per 1,000 women per year (this was "the benefit"), but an increase by 2.8 cases of life-threatening side effects from tamoxifen, such as uterine cancer, blood clots, and stroke. There was no difference in the overall survival rates in either group. It's important, too, to keep in mind that the benefit of tamoxifen applied only to women in this particular study, who were believed to have twice the risk of breast cancer. So, women with a lower risk of breast cancer will benefit less.

Although it was found that there were fewer cases of breast cancer in the women taking tamoxifen compared to the women on a placebo, we don't know if tamoxifen prevented breast cancer from occurring or if the cancers were delayed and will appear later. That's because this study was too short to assess whether longer exposure to tamoxifen can cause other types of cancer to develop or whether breast cancer rates might increase after women stopped taking the drug. In Europe, there are two ongoing studies with tamoxifen in women with a high risk of breast cancer. These studies have shown no difference in the number of breast cancer cases between the women who took tamoxifen and those who took a placebo.

The Breast Cancer Study also showed that the breast cancers that developed in women using tamoxifen were also the easiest ones to treat: small tumours and those that were estrogen-receptor positive (i.e. the cell thrives on estrogen). Therefore, taking tamoxifen does not guarantee that if breast cancer occurs it will be diagnosed an early stage, and it does not affect your survival. But taking tamoxifen for five years can delay the appearance of breast cancer and may decrease the number of tumours that will develop.

Much of the misinformation about what tamoxifen supposedly does occurs in the media. For example, the television show *The Lehrer NewsHour* presented a segment on February 18, 1999, stating that tamoxifen prevented breast cancer. Corrections were made on-air and to the PBS Web site March 22, 1999, after letters of complaint and protest were sent to PBS by scientists who made it clear that the results of the tamoxifen study did *not* prove, in any way, that the drug could prevent breast cancer.

The use of tamoxifen as a prevention therapy is extremely controversial because tamoxifen is an anti-estrogen drug, which means that it has side effects when given to healthy women without any sign of breast cancer, and these side effects need to be weighed against the perceived benefits of the drug. The Breast Cancer Study revealed that life-threatening risks of tamoxifen include: endometrial or uterine cancer (this occurs at a rate of 2–7 times greater in tamoxifen-treated women, and earlier studies show that tamoxifen-related endometrial cancer can be more severe than other forms of endometrial cancer); blood clot in the lungs; blood clot in the veins; stroke; liver cancer or liver problems.

Other side effects of tamoxifen include hot flashes, vaginal discharge or bleeding, menstrual irregularities, cataracts, colour blindness, and changes in vision. Hair loss and skin rashes have also been reported, and 15 per cent of women in the Breast Cancer Study stopped using the drug because of side effects.

Supporters of tamoxifen argue that although the incidence of uterine cancer doubled in the study, since uterine cancer is curable, and breast cancer isn't, one is the lesser evil and worth the risk. However, 1997 research presented at the World Conference on Breast Cancer and the Environment, held in Kingston, Ontario, revealed that tamoxifen also increases risk of ovarian and cervical cancer, and can also cause depression.

critics of the breast cancer study

Critics of this study argue that the women participants were not informed of the risks tamoxifen carried below the waist, such as menopausal symptoms, endometrial and liver cancer. The study's recruitment criteria was also criticized; 98.2 per cent of all women recruited were white, affecting any meaningful data for women of other ethnic origins. In addition, the drug has not been tested in women with less than 10 years to live; with a prior history of breast cancer, or in whom breast cancer of any type was suspected; with a history of any other cancer diagnosed less than 10 years ago; with existing diseases in which tamoxifen would be dangerous, such as diabetes or heart disease.; on hormone replacement therapy (women with an intact uterus), unopposed estrogen therapy (women who have had a hysterectomy), on oral contraceptives or male hormones. The drug has also not been tested on women who already took tamoxifen; those with history of macular degeneration (eye problems); and those who refused to undergo regular sampling of their endometrial tissue.

Critics also argue that the Breast Cancer Study was rooted in profit. When tamoxifen is touted as a "prevention drug," then, in theory, one half of the female population becomes the target market. And that means someone will make a lot of money off of women's fears over breast cancer, even though there wasn't clear proof that tamoxifen can prevent breast cancer in healthy women who show no signs of the disease.

Research ethicists challenge the Breast Cancer Study on ethical grounds, stating that tamoxifen is not suitable as a prevention drug in pre-symptomatic women because it is not "relatively safe" or "free from life-threatening side effects"; it should be administered to women *clearly* at risk for this disease rather than to women who merely exhibit superficial risk markers, such as age or race; risk factors of the disease "should be well-understood" prior to undertaking such a study; and the drug should be proven effective for preventing breast cancer.

Finally, critics maintain that while tamoxifen is not many things, it is also not a *primary* prevention; it serves to further medicate healthy women instead of addressing lifestyle or behaviour changes that can reduce *exposure* to known carcinogens or mutagens. Essentially, tamoxifen is seen by many as a wolf in sheep's clothing; it is aggressive treatment that is called "prevention."

As of this writing, Public Citizen, an organization founded by consumer advocate Ralph Nader, and the National Women's Health Network issued to the FDA a Citizen's Petition to Revise the Labelling on Tamoxifen. Much of the information in this section was taken from the groups' proposed medication guide for patients. The guide was proposed because both groups felt that the current FDA-approved label provides inadequate information and is difficult for both patients and physicians to interpret.

preventative mastectomy

Doctors sometimes recommend preventative or prophylactic mastectomy. Surgeons I've interviewed tell me that when it comes to this procedure, it's the patient who wants it rather than the doctor. While this procedure does lower your risk, it doesn't guarantee that you'll never get breast cancer. In any event, the only scenarios where preventive mastectomy should ever be considered are as follows:

- Risk of bilateral, premenopausal familial breast cancer. For example, if your mother and sister both developed bilateral invasive breast cancer at, say, age 35, you would be considered very likely to develop breast cancer around this age, too.
- Diagnosis of lobular carcinoma in situ (a marker for breast cancer risk) is considered a sign of higher cancer risk in either breast. Depending on your age, medical and family history, preventative mastectomy may be an option.
- Breast cancer has been diagnosed in one breast. Depending on the staging and invasiveness of the cancer, a preventative mastectomy for the other breast may be an option.

The decision to have a preventative mastectomy is highly individual. With the advent of far more sensitive mammograms, which will presumably get more sensitive as time goes on, many experts are abandoning preventative mastectomy as a prevention strategy. So if this procedure is being recommended, you should definitely seek out a second opinion from a breast surgeon, not just a general surgeon.

A double preventive, or prophylactic mastectomy (also called a bilateral prophylactic mastectomy) lowers your risk of breast cancer by 90 per cent, but cannot guarantee that you will never get breast cancer, because some breast tissue remains.

new advances

"Breakthrough treatments" or possible prevention therapies for breast cancer explode into medical journals, newspapers, and television news reports daily. Did you hear about the drug faslodex, which is considered to be more powerful and effective than tamoxifen—in a test tube, that is! There is also promising news about a technique that combines magnetic resonance imaging (MRI) and lasers, which can zap breast tumours on the spot. (But who will pay for this equipment to make it standard therapy? Ever heard of budgets?)

The three questions you must always ask when you read or hear about new treatments and therapies for breast cancer are:

1. *Is the treatment experimental or readily available?* Unless the treatment is readily available, it means that many more studies, clinical trials, and experiments need to be done before the treatment is offered by your doctor. Or, it may mean that the therapy is so expensive, no average woman with breast cancer can possibly afford it, let alone the government, and so it will not become standard therapy without years of lobbying and activism.
2. *Is the new treatment of the week proven to work in lots of women who actually had (have) breast cancer, or is the hype based on animal studies or clinical trials involving a ridiculously small sample of, say, five women in a suburb?* In other words, when something works in a small sample of women, there could be dozens of reasons for the drug's success that have nothing to do with the drug itself, and more to do with the small sample of women (lifestyle, diet, and so on).
3. *When will the drug be approved or available?* How many times have you read in the newspaper or heard on the news the famous last words of a hyped report?: "...but scientists say the drug is years away from approval" or "Critics of the drug say many more studies are needed to prove its safety and effectiveness." Start paying more attention to the last sentence of the article or report than the headline. Headlines that start with "Promising New Therapy for Breast Cancer" usually end with a "But..."

what to eat

Your greatest protection from breast cancer is to modify your diet. A heart-smart diet (see chapter 2), combined with a colon-friendly diet (see chapter 5) are considered "breast cancer protection" diets. By lowering the fat content in our diets, we lower the amount of fat-soluble toxins that live in our bodies. Also, the more fat we eat, the bigger our fat cells get, and the more estrogen our fat cells make—considered a risk factor for breast cancer, too. Because breast cancer is also linked to environmental chemicals, you may wish to choose organic produce.

eating less toxic foods

To cut down on dietary pollutants that can increase the risk of breast cancer, cut down on:

- Meat. Most livestock is fed hormones, which we ingest. Even organically raised meat, such as free-range chicken, can still be exposed to pesticides (which may contain estrogenic mimics), in the vegetation *they* ingest, which can wind up inside our own bodies, contributing to an estrogen overload. Meat is also higher in fat. (Since we're omnivores, however, our bodies are meant to eat a certain amount of meat and other animal products, good sources of iron, vitamin B_{12}, and zinc.)
- Animal products, such as eggs.
- Fish. If the fish you eat is from contaminated waters, you may be ingesting mercury or PCBs, which gets stored in your fat. Otherwise, fish that is contaminant-free is quite healthy.

Before you eat, ask some questions about the food you consume. You can find out what your animal produce has eaten, and whether it was injected with anything by calling Agriculture and Agrafood Canada at 613-952-8000. (and in the U.S., the United States Department of Agriculture, USDA, at 202-720-2791.) By contacting these agencies, you can also find out what waters your fish has swum in and what substances your grown produce was sprayed with.

You can find "safe food" that is organically grown through a number of natural produce supermarkets and through organizations like Canadian Organic Growers (COG). To find out more about your supermarket's produce-buying habits contact the store's head office.

plant chemicals (a.ka. phytochemicals) that can protect your breasts

Studies show that many phytochemicals can reduce the risk of breast cancer. Consider the following:

- Algin. Found in brown kelp (also known as kombu or laminaria, often used as a wrap (e.g., sushi) and food seasoning in soups and salads
- Bioflavonoids. Found in fresh fruits, vegetables, and other greens, especially deeply coloured produce like orange squash and blueberries
- Carotenoids. Found in apricots (including dried), carrots, collard greens, kale, spinach, sweet potatoes, tomatoes, pumpkin, watermelon
- Fibre. Found in all organic whole grains, fruits, vegetables
- Flavonoids. Found in deeply coloured fruits, especially blueberries, huckleberries, oranges, lemons, strawberries, green and red peppers, broccoli
- Indole 3-carbinol. Found in cruciferous vegetables, like broccoli, cabbage, cauliflower
- Phytoestrogens. Found in soy products
- Selenium. Found in brewer's yeast, garlic, organic whole grains, safe seafood (tuna, shellfish); supplements combining selenium with garlic work synergistically
- Sulfur-rich amino acids. Found in garlic
- Sulforaphane. Found in bok choy, broccoli, cauliflower
- Vitamin C. Found in broccoli, cauliflower, citrus fruits, peppers
- Tocopherols. Found in vegetable oils, almonds, soybeans, sunflower seeds, wheat germ and wheat germ oil

immune boosters

Immune boosters stimulate the immune system or strengthen it to help fight diseases such as cancer. Today, many substances, such as echinacea and zinc, are as popular as vitamin C. Here's an overview of some of the well-known ones:

- Echinacea. This is a flower that belongs to the sunflower family. It's believed that echinacea increases the number of cells in your immune system to fight off disease.
- Essiac. This is a mixture of four herbs comprising Indian rhubarb, sheepshead sorrel, slippery elm, and burdock root. Essiac is believed to

strengthen the immune system, improve appetite, supply essential nutrients to the body, possibly relieve pain, and ultimately, prolong life.

- Ginseng. This is a root used in Chinese medicine, but it's believed to enhance the immune system and boost the activity of white blood cells.
- Green Tea. This is a popular Asian tea made from a plant called *Camellia sinensis*. The active chemical in green tea is epigallocatechin gallate (EGCG). It is believed that green tea neutralizes free radicals, which are carcinogenic. It is considered to be an anti-cancer tea, particularly for stomach, lung, and skin cancers.
- Iscador (a.k.a. mistletoe). Iscador is made through a fermentation process using different kinds of mistletoe, a plant known for its white berries. More popular as an anti-tumour treatment in Europe, it's believed that iscador works by enhancing the immune system and inhibiting tumour growth.
- Paul d'Arco (a.k.a. taheebo). This usually comes in the form of a tea made from the inner bark of a tree called tabebuia. It's believed to be a cleansing agent, can be used as an antimicrobial agent, and is said to stop tumour growth.
- Wheatgrass. This is grass grown from wheatberry seeds, which is rich in chlorophyll. Its juice contains more than 100 vitamins, minerals, and nutrients, and is believed to contain a number of cancer-fighting and immune-boosting properties.

The following spices are considered to be anti-cancer agents. Use some of the spices on this list in your next meal:

- Garlic
- Tumeric
- Onions
- Black pepper
- Asfetida
- Pippali
- Cumin and poppy seeds
- Kandathiipile
- Neem flowers
- Mananthakkali, drumstick and basil leaves
- Ponnakanni
- Parsley

how to move

By following the guidelines under How To Move in chapters 2 and 3, you can help lower your risk of breast cancer. In addition, deep-breathing exercises can help to stimulate both oxygen flow and your immune system. And try the stretching exercises outlined at the end of this chapter. The best movements of all when it comes to breast health is to feel your breasts for changes or lumps.

breast self-examination (BSE)

This method should be called "get to know your breasts." It involves specific steps of feeling your breast at the same time each month and distinguishing suspicious lumps from normal lumpy/bumpy breasts. In addition, you can't know if a lump has remained unchanged unless you've been checking your breasts monthly.

While you're still menstruating, you'll need to do a BSE after your period ends when your breasts are least tender and lumpy. When you're pregnant, BSE should be done monthly throughout all stages of your pregnancy. When you're breast-feeding, perform BSE on a monthly basis after a feeding, when your breasts aren't filled with milk. And then, after your periods return, perform BSE after a feeding, *after* your period. If you're past menopause, just pick the same time each month, like the first or fifteenth of the month, to do it.

Although the steps to BSE are outlined below, make sure your doctor or health care practitioner shows you how to do it as well. In addition, there is a kit available through the National Cancer Institute called the *Mammacare Learning System*. The kit was developed at the University of Florida, and was partially funded by the National Cancer Institute. It consists of a 45-minute video and a 30-page instructional manual. This kit was designed to teach you how to do a breast self-exam using a "vertical grid pattern." currently the most effective pattern.

the steps to BSE

1. *Visually inspect your breasts*. Stand in front of the mirror and look closely at your breasts. You're looking for dimpling, puckering (like an orange peel in appearance), or noticeable lumps. Do you see any discharge that dribbles out on its own or bleeding from the nipple? Any funny dry patches on the nipple?

2. *Visually inspect your breasts with your arms raised.* Now, raise your arms over your head and in front of the mirror, and look for the same things. Raising your arms smooths out the breast a little more so changes are more obvious.
3. *Palpation* (feeling your breast). Lie down on the bed with a pillow under your left shoulder and place your left hand under your head. With the flat part of the fingertips of your right hand, examine your left breast for a lump, using a gentle circular motion. Imagine that the breast is a clock, and make sure you feel each "hour," as well as the nipple area and armpit area.
4. *Repeat step 3, but reverse sides, examining your right breast with your left hand.*
5. *If you find a lump...* Note the size, shape, and how painful it is. A suspicious lump is usually painless, about 1/4–1/2 inch in size, and remains unchanged from month to month. Get the lump looked at as soon as you can, or if you're comfortable doing so, wait for the next cycle/month. If the lump changes in the next cycle by shrinking or becoming painful, it's not cancerous, but should be looked at anyway. If the suspicious lump stays the same, definitely get it looked at as soon as possible. Keep in mind that breast cysts are common, variable in size, and occasionally tender.
6. *If discharge oozes out of your nipple on its own, or if blood comes out...* see your doctor immediately. Don't wait.
7. *If your nipple is dry and patchy...* see your doctor immediately. Don't wait.

stretches good for your breasts

1. Chest Expander: Stand with feet hip width apart, arms resting comfortably at your sides. Gently allow your arms to drift backward, until you can clasp your hands behind you. Exhale, keeping your body aligned while you stretch your arms behind you. Breathe deeply and hold (see figure i).
2. Cobra (Upward-Facing Dog): Lie on your belly with your palms down and adjacent to your shoulders. Slowly raise your upper body, lifting all but the lower abdomen toward the ceiling. Breathe deeply. Release.
3. Child's Pose: Sit on your heels. Bring your forehead to the floor in front of you. Breathe into the back of the rib cage, feeling the stretch in your spine. Hold as long as it's comfortable.

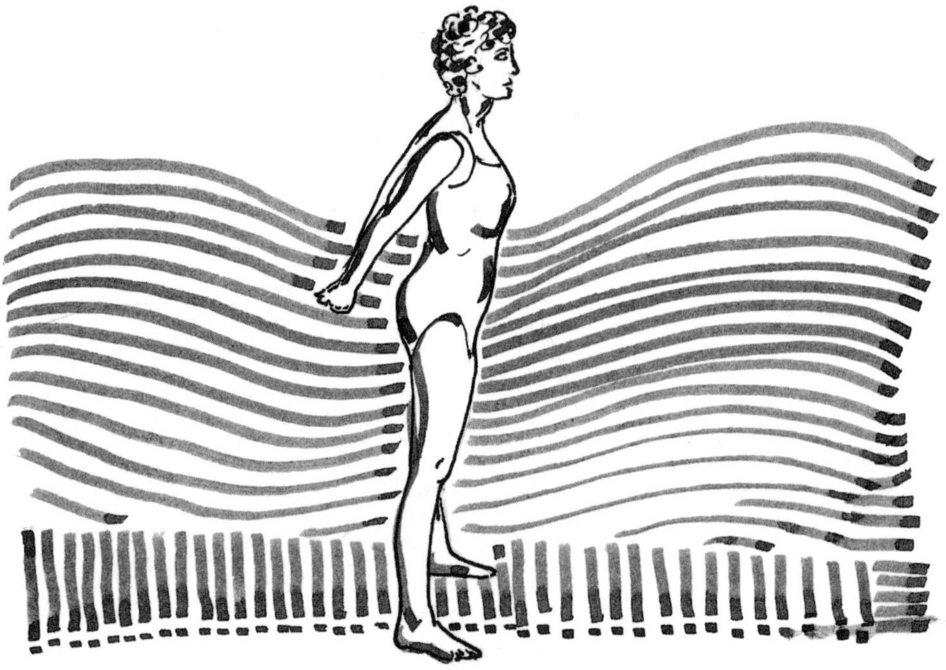

figure i

4. Surrender Squeeze: Clasp your hands in front of you as if in prayer. Slowly move your hands backward to squeeze your shoulder blades together. Hold for 10 seconds, breathing deeply.
5. Neurolymphatic points for Breast Pain and Chest Soreness: The lymphatics are tiny vessels that carry waste products from the body's peripherals to the neck area, where they empty into the veins leading to the heart. Massage each point deeply and firmly for 30 seconds.

five

colon health

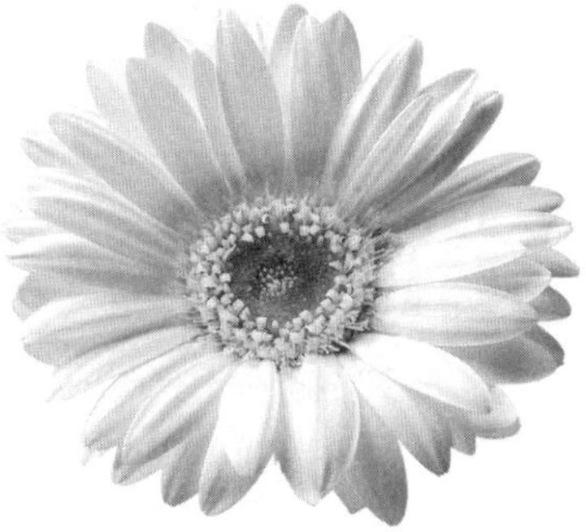

Keeping your colon healthy is the key to avoiding a number of health problems from head to toe, including obesity, heart disease, a variety of cancers, including, of course, colon and rectal cancer. Many women don't realize that colon cancer strikes slightly more women than men, especially beyond the age of 45. And many women don't realize that colon cancer is almost 90 per cent preventable through diet, exercise, and regular screenings.

staying regular

The colon essentially acts as a solid-waste container, drying out the waste that doesn't get absorbed farther up. The nervous system controls the muscular contractions of the colon, which slowly move waste downward, toward the rectum. We experience these stronger muscular contractions as "the urge." And once we feel the urge, we sit down, relax, and allow the gentle contractions to overtake us. All we have to do is relax and the anal sphincter will open to allow the passage of stool.

The frequency of bowel movements varies from person to person. Although many North American sources say it's normal to move your bowels anywhere from a few times a day to a few times a week, if you're not having one to three large, bulky, soft but firm bowel movements daily, you probably have a tendency to be constipated. A normal stool is solid or "formed" but not hard, and certainly should not contain mucus or blood. The stools should pass without cramps, pain, or strain. However, normal stools can pass noisily, since natural gas (called flatus)—swallowed air (nitrogen) that gets trapped in the lower intestine—often comes out with the stools, or independently.

constipation

Constipation means that you are not experiencing an urge to move your bowels, and when you do, the stools are hard and difficult to pass. Generally, if more than three days have passed since your last bowel movement, the stools will harden. The colon will continue to dry out the stools because that's what colons do.

Most constipation is "functional" in that there is no disease or organic problem at work; it's a lifestyle problem, having to do with ignoring the urge to go, or not allowing enough time in the morning to create the urge to go by drinking or eating something. If you ignore the urge too often, you may stop feeling an urge altogether. Studies comparing bowel habits of North Americans to Africans show that the incidence of colon cancer is higher in North Americans, who have less frequent bowel movements than Africans. We can learn from these studies, and modify our lifestyles accordingly. The idea is to find a happy medium, because chronic diarrhea is also dangerous to your health. In fact, it's far more troublesome than chronic constipation.

By simply obeying your urges, you can avoid constipation. Learning to suppress the urge to defecate can create what is called a "lazy bowel." When you feel the urge to defecate, drop what you're doing and get to the toilet. We all know ways of excusing ourselves to make or take "important calls." Why not make your nature call the most important call of your day?

Another way to obey the nature call is to give yourself enough time to receive the call in the first place. If you get out of bed, get dressed, and rush out the door immediately, you may be one of millions who suffers from "commuter constipation."

If constipation is a more sudden or recent occurrence in your life, there could be other causes, such as:

- Hypothyroidism (low-functioning thyroid). Request a thyroid stimulating hormone test (TSH) to check for thyroid function, if you suspect this.
- Pregnancy or changes in the menstrual cycle. It's not unusual for women to experience constipation at these times.
- Hot weather. When you're perspiring, and losing body fluid, you could become constipated.
- Stress. This is often the cause.
- Travel. Changes in schedule, diet, and time zones can interfere with regularity.
- Anal sores (includes fissures, hemorrhoids, or herpes).
- Medications (particularly pain control medications in chronic illness).
- Periods of vomiting and diarrhea.

chronic constipation

Chronic constipation can be caused by a variety of things, including laxative abuse, diseases affecting body tissues, nerve or muscle control, inflammation, scarring or blockage in the lower intestine; spinal injuries; prolonged bedrest or being bedridden. Again, lack of exercise and poor diet are the most common causes of chronic constipation. (See What to Eat and How to Move at the end of this chapter for helpful suggestions.)

hemorrhoids

The straining caused by chronic constipation can lead to hemorrhoids. These are swollen blood vessels or veins around the anus either inside (internal) covered by the inner lining, or protruding from the rectum. A classic symptom of internal hemorrhoids is finding bright red blood squirting into the toilet water, covering your stool, on toilet paper, or in the toilet bowl. Sometimes an internal hemorrhoid is large enough that it protrudes through your rectum, and hangs outside the body, known as a *protruding hemorrhoid*. Since bleeding is a problem with internal hemorrhoids, you can become anemic.

To find some relief, try warm tub or sitz baths, when the water just covers your hips, several times a day. Don't use anything in the water except a little baking soda (optional), and don't stay in longer than about 10 minutes.

Stool softeners may help you pass stool more comfortably, while ice packs will help reduce swelling (10 minutes on/10 minutes off). Frequently shifting your positions while standing or sitting is also helpful. Over-the-counter hemorrhoid medication can provide relief as well, but won't shrink the hemorrhoid. If the problem is not resolving itself, the hemorrhoid can be removed in your doctor's office.

the trouble with laxatives

The best way to know the right laxatives is to know the *wrong* ones. Avoid anything that is a *stimulant laxative*, which can include herbal laxatives, such as senna and cascara sagrada. There is some debate regarding the latter, however. Many herbalists maintain that cascara sagrada, unlike senna, is more a tonic than a laxative, does not to create a dependency, and in fact, may be helpful for your colon. However, like other stimulant laxatives, it works by stimulating the colon to contract, creating a bowel movement and, with too much use, a dependency. The medical expert for this book strongly advises against using cascara sagrada. A dependency on laxatives means that you will not be able to move your bowels without the laxative because your colon becomes used to it. There are several herbal teas and concoctions that promote digestion and regularity through the use of harmless spices or ingredients. See What To Eat at the end of this chapter for details.

If you must take an occasional laxative, the best kind are bulking agents, which are sold as laxatives but are actually not a laxative per se. Metamucil® is an example of a bulking agent. Adopting a water-with-fibre routine (see What To Eat) will probably cure you of constipation. Try that first before you try a laxative. If nothing is working, and you haven't moved your bowels in five or six days, insert a glycerein suppository overnight, and in the morning things should get moving. If there's still no action, the next step is to try an enema, and after that, a mild laxative, such as milk of magnesia. If you are still constipated after trying various options, you may have a bowel obstruction of some sort, which a gastroenterologist can diagnose and treat.

retraining your colon

For many, years of ignoring the urge to defecate, and laxative dependency, has made it impossible to "go it alone." Take heart: you can train your bowel to recapture its youth. Here's the recipe: drink a glass of warm water in the morning as soon as you wake up, and insert a glycerein suppository, then move around a bit (make your bed, do some stretches, etc.) for about 3 or 4 minutes. Sit on the toilet and gently push for about two minutes. If nothing happens, get up and leave. If you practice this routine every day for 3–6 months, you should be able to train your colon to have a bowel movement when you drink warm water in the morning. In other words, the warm water will stimulate your colon. Missing even a day of this routine could set you back weeks, though!

bowel diseases

Bowel diseases can plague women of all ages, but they can become aggravated as we age. This section addresses two common bowel conditions that affect women: irritable bowel syndrome and inflammatory bowel disease.

irritable bowel syndrome (IBS)

A most confusing label has come into vogue, which defines the bowel habits of between 25–55 million North Americans, two-thirds of whom are women. The label is *irritable bowel syndrome* (IBS), which refers to unusual bowel "patterns" that alternate between diarrhea and constipation, and everything in between. IBS is also referred to as irritable or spastic colon; spastic, mucus, nervous, laxative, cathartic or functional colitis; spastic bowel; nervous indigestion; functional dyspepsia; pylorospasm; and functional bowel disease. The problem with using the word "irritable" is that irritation is *not* what's going on. It also sounds too much like "inflammatory," which is not what's going on, either. Worse, many family doctors will say "IBS" instead of "We don't know what's going on—but have you tried fibre?"

The term "irritable" bowel syndrome came into use to describe a bowel that is overly sensitive to normal activity. In other words, when the nerve endings that line the bowel are too sensitive, the nerves controlling the gastrointestinal tract can become overactive, making the bowel overly responsive or "irritable" to normal things, such as passing gas or fluid. In other words, the bowel may want to pass a stool before it's time. The bowel, in a sense, becomes too "touchy" for comfort. However, since we tend to think of irritable, when used clinically, as something that is red, irritated, or inflamed, this label is more confusing than defining. IBS has nothing to do with irritation, inflammation, or any organic disease process. It has to do with nerves.

The term IBS also implies that a diagnosis of your symptoms has been made and there is a definite cause—and cure—for your condition. This is not so at all. IBS is a diagnosis made in the absence of any other diagnosis. There is no test to confirm IBS; only tests to rule out other causes for your symptoms. The term functional bowel disorder is beginning to catch on instead of IBS, because functional means that there is no disease. Yet no matter what you call it, roughly half of all digestive disorders are attributed to IBS.

After the common cold, IBS is the chief cause of absenteeism. Many doctors compare IBS to asthma in that there are a number of causes with the same outcome: asthma may be related to allergies, or a hundred other things; similarly, IBS has many different causes that are difficult to pin down. However, stress and dietary factors are the chief causes.

IBS symptoms

IBS symptoms are characterized by frequent, violent episodes of diarrhea which will almost always strike around a stressful situation. Over 60 per cent of IBS sufferers report that their symptoms first coincided with stressful life events, while 40–60 per cent of people with IBS also suffer from anxiety disorders or depression, compared to 20 per cent of people with other gastrointestinal disorders. Stressful life events that can bring on IBS include death of a loved one, separation and divorce, unresolved conflict or grief, moving to a new city or job, as well as a history of physical or sexual abuse in childhood. People often experience IBS symptoms before job interviews or plane trips.

Many IBS sufferers find that their symptoms persist well beyond the stressful life event, and the episodes will invade their normal routine. There need not be one single stressful event that precipitates IBS; it could first present itself after you've been in a stressful job over a long period of time or subjected to the normal stresses of modern life for a long period of time.

The episodes of diarrhea that characterize IBS are often accompanied by crampy, abdominal pains or gas, which are relieved by a bowel movement. The pain may shift around in the abdomen as well. After the diarrhea episodes, you may be plagued by long bouts of constipation, or the feeling that you're not emptying your bowels completely when you do go to the bathroom. Again, IBS refers to an irregular bowel *pattern* rather than one particular episode. The pattern is that there is no *normal* pattern of bowel movements; it is often one extreme or the other.

Your stools may also contain mucus, which can make the stool long and ropelike or wormlike. The mucus is normally secreted by the colon to help the stool along in a normal movement. In IBS, your colon secretes too much mucus.

Blood mixed with your stools means "This is *not* IBS, but something else." Some people may also suffer from diarrhea alone, or gas and constipation alone. Other symptoms include bloating, nausea, and loss of appetite. Fever, weight loss, or severe pain is not a sign of IBS but of some other disorder.

Many people find it confusing that IBS can cause both constipation and diarrhea, two conditions which seem to be at opposite ends of the spectrum. What happens is that instead of the slow muscular contractions that normally move the bowels, spasms occur, which can either result in an explosion or a blockage. Akin to a sudden gust of wind, it can blow the door wide open (diarrhea), or blow it shut (constipation); it all depends on the direction of the wind at the time.

It's important to note the timing of your diarrhea; in IBS, your sleep should not be disturbed by it. The episodes will always occur either after a meal or in the early evening.

What distinguishes IBS from infectious diarrhea or inflammatory bowel diseases are: finding relief through defecation; noticing looser stools when the bowel movement is precipitated by pain; noticing more frequent bowel movements when you experience pain; noticing abdominal bloating or distention; noticing mucus in the stools; and feeling that you have not completely emptied your bowels.

what to rule out

As mentioned above, the symptoms of IBS can be signs of many other problems. Therefore, before you accept a diagnosis of IBS, make sure your doctor has taken a careful history to investigate:

- Dietary culprits, food allergies, lactose intolerance, or just plain poor diet—high fats/starch; low fibre
- Intestinal bacterial, viral, or parasitic infections (Where have you travelled lately? What are your sexual habits?)
- Overgrowth of *C. difficile*, a common cause of infectious diarrhea
- Yeast in the gastrointestinal tract, called candidiasis, which is notorious for causing IBS symptoms (eating yogurt every day should clear this up)
- Medications

- Gastrointestinal disorders, such as dysmotility, where the stomach muscles are not moving properly, causing bloating, nausea, and other problems
- Enzyme deficiencies (the pancreas may not be secreting enough enzymes to break down your food)
- Serious disease such as inflammatory bowel disease (IBS) or signs of cancer.

stress and IBS

It's possible to have a pristine diet, rule out all forms of organic disease, yet still suffer from IBS while under stress. In the same way that you can sweat, blush, or cry under emotional stress, your gastrointestinal tract may also react to stress by "weeping"—producing excessive water and mucus, overreacting to normal stimuli such as eating. What often happens, however, is that there is a delayed gut reaction to stress, and you may not experience IBS symptoms until your stress has passed.

Apparently, under stress the brain becomes more active as a defence. For example, when we're running away from a predator, we have to think quickly and act quickly, so our heart rates increase, we sweat more, and so on. During this defensive mode, the entire nervous system can become exaggerated; that's what causes "butterflies in the stomach." The nerves controlling the gastrointestinal tract therefore become highly sensitive, which can cause IBS symptoms. Studies show, for example, that IBS symptoms are more common on weekday mornings than afternoons or weekends, and IBS symptoms do not appear at night while you're sleeping.

women and IBS

Why is IBS more common in women? For one thing, women menstruate, and experience normal mood fluctuations related to their natural menstrual cycles. As women reach menopause, and the cycle becomes more erratic, so, too, can the bowel, as it can be stimulated by uterine contractions. The first day of a woman's period is often a day during which she has several loose bowel movements. (A common symptom of labour is diarrhea and vomiting. This occurs because of the intensity of uterine contractions, which create ripples throughout the gastrointestinal tract.)

Finally, women are much more prone to eating disorders and laxative abuse, as well as domestic abuse, resulting in continuous emotional upset and stress, all of which wreak havoc on the gastrointestinal tract.

inflammatory bowel disease

Inflammatory bowel disease (IBD) is a serious, chronic condition that can be life-threatening in extreme cases. IBD means that one or more parts of your small or large intestine is inflamed, causing symptoms that range from unpleasant but manageable, to severe and debilitating.

When inflammation and/or ulceration is confined to the inner lining of the colon (*colitis*) and rectum (*proctitis*), you have what's known as *ulcerative colitis*, which is confined to the colon and not the small bowel. The inflammation will usually start in the rectum and may spread throughout the colon. Because it's inflamed, the colon will not be able to do what it was designed to do: hold your solid waste. As a result, it will need to empty waste as soon as it receives it; you'll experience this as diarrhea. The inflammation will cause the cells that line the colon to slough off or die, causing open sores, or ulcers, to form on the lining, which could then form pus or mucus. So the diarrhea is often tinged with blood, pus, or mucus.

When the inflammation goes beyond the lining into the actual walls of the intestine, you have what's known as *Crohn's disease*, which usually attacks a part of the gastrointestinal tract (GI tract) above the colon, in the ileum, the third and last part of the small intestine. For this reason, Crohn's disease is also known as ileitis or regional enteritis. But Crohn's disease can also attack the colon and/or other parts of the GI tract.

If your intestines were a trench coat, ulcerative colitis would be confined to the lining of the coat below the belt, or ileum; that is, the lining of the colon and rectum. Crohn's disease would affect the entire coat starting at the belt, and possibly all the way up to the collar (the upper GI tract). Or it could start at the belt and affect everything below it (the lower GI tract). Think of the belt as the official separation between the upper and lower GI tract.

The risk of colon cancer is about 32 times higher if you have ulcerative colitis. That's because ulcerative colitis can cause the cells that line the colon to become precancerous, known as *dysplasia*. If only the rectum or lower part of the colon is involved, then your risk is not any higher than in the general population.

Nevertheless, if you've had ulcerative colitis for more than eight years, you should be screened annually for evidence of dysplasia through sigmoidoscopy or colonoscopy (see page 137). Tissue biopsies can be obtained through colonoscopy. If dysplasia is found, you may be offered the option of a colectomy, surgical removal of the colon, to prevent the spread of precancerous cells and the development of full-blown colon cancer.

ulcerative colitis

You may have ulcerative colitis, and be at an increased risk of colon cancer, but never have been officially diagnosed with this condition. Abdominal cramps combined with bloody diarrhea, which could contain mucus and/or pus, and frequent, urgent bowel movements are the most common symptoms of ulcerative colitis. The diarrhea usually strikes immediately after meals or at night. Some people may also lose control of their bowel movements (fecal incontinence) or pass stool in the belief that it is just gas. Obviously, these symptoms can interfere with many daily activities, including sleep. Not all people will suffer from severe symptoms; the severity depends on where the inflammation is located. Sometimes it's confined to the rectum, or one side of the colon, as opposed to the entire colon.

When symptoms *are* severe, you can suffer from all of the following: fatigue; weight loss; loss of appetite and/or nausea; rectal bleeding; malnutrition, mainly due to the loss of fluids and nutrients; and anemia, from bleeding.

The same causes that trigger the immune system to attack bowel tissue can also cause it to attack other body tissues, causing what's known as "complications" such as skin lesions, arthritis, inflammation of the eyes, or liver disorders, including jaundice and cirrhosis, which could necessitate a liver transplant.

In severe but rare cases, the colon enlarges and distends, known as *toxic megacolon*. This condition will cause fever, abdominal pain, dehydration, and malnutrition. In this case, surgery is necessary to prevent the colon from rupturing.

Crohn's disease

The symptoms of Crohn's disease are similar to those that indicate ulcerative colitis: abdominal cramps and diarrhea, resulting in rectal bleeding, anemia, weight loss, and fever (fever is not usually a symptom in ulcerative colitis unless the colon enlarges). The fever makes it easy to confuse Crohn's disease with infectious diarrhea. The location of the abdominal cramping in Crohn's disease is usually in the lower right side.

Because Crohn's disease attacks the intestinal walls and can occur higher up the GI tract, obstruction can take place due to narrowing of passageways, which swell and develop scar tissue. Fistulas, "ulcer tunnels" between tissues, can develop around the bladder, rectum, anus, or vagina. These tunnels can become infected and filled with pus. They are a common complication and often are associated with pockets of infection or abscesses (infected areas of pus).

As with ulcerative colitis, the autoimmune nature of Crohn's disease can also cause other body parts to inflame, including joints, skin, eyes, and mouth. Kidney stones and gallstones are a further complication of Crohn's.

getting an accurate diagnosis

Since the symptoms of both ulcerative colitis and Crohn's disease are virtually indistinguishable, the only way to get an accurate diagnosis is to have a doctor examine your bowel tissue under a microscope. This is done by a pathologist (a doctor who specializes in analyzing tissue specimens under a microscope). There are even pathologists who subspecialize in gastroenterology. A GI specialist can get a tissue sample through sigmoidoscopy or colonoscopy.

Your doctor will also want to collect a stool sample to rule out infections or parasites, which can also cause mucus or pus-tinged diarrhea. And finally, blood tests will confirm whether you're anemic or have a high white blood cell count, which is a sign of inflammation.

screening for colon cancer

Colorectal cancer—cancer in the colon and/or rectum—accounts for roughly 13 per cent of all cancers, and is considered the second leading cause of cancer deaths, next to lung cancer. Colorectal cancer develops from an earlier growth known as a polyp. It is important to note that all colon cancer comes from polyps; but not all polyps become colon cancer. What this means is that by screening for polyps on a regular basis, you can "catch" colon cancer before it ever develops. Think of polyps screening, or polyps hunting, as the Pap test for colon cancer. In the same way that most women will be spared a diagnosis of cervical cancer thanks to the Pap test, most people who go for regular polyp screening should be spared a diagnosis of colon cancer. (The screening procedure may also detect other diseases of the lower intestine, such as ulcerative colitis.)

Even if you are diagnosed with colorectal cancer, it's important to keep in mind that colorectal cancers develop in glandular tissue, but are considered very treatable when caught in an early stage.

Colon cancer can also be preventable through diet. Of all the studies done on cancer and dietary fat, the strongest connections can be made between high-fat diets and colon cancer. In other words, people who consume high quantities of fat have higher rates of colon cancer; people who consume low quantities of fat have lower rates of colon cancer.

As for fibre, studies show that people who consume high quantities of fibre have lower rates of colon cancer, while people who consume low quantities of fibre have higher rates of colon cancer. In addition, people who have regular bowel movements experience lower incidences of colon cancer than people who are chronically constipated. (See What To Eat at the end of this chapter for details.)

screening guidelines

Anyone age 45 or older is at an increased risk for colorectal cancer, although occasionally it occurs in people who are in their 30s. In the general population, 1 in 20 people without any known risk factors for colorectal cancer will develop it.

Known risk factors for colorectal cancer include a history of ulcerative colitis; a family history of colorectal cancer; a history of benign tumours (polyps) in the colon or rectum; a diet high in fat and low in fibre; and possibly a family history of breast or ovarian cancers, but this is hotly debated. Annual screening is recommended by age 45, or even younger.

No matter how old you are, or how recently you've been screened for evidence of colon cancer, there are certain red-flag symptoms that warrant immediate investigation by a specialist, called either a colorectal surgeon or a gastroenterologist. The word that characterizes alarming symptoms from chronic symptoms is "sudden." If you're between 45 and 55, and you suddenly notice the onset of any of the following symptoms, don't wait and see what happens; get yourself to a doctor's office as soon as possible, where you can be referred for testing to a specialist.

- Changes in bowel habits
- Changes in stool consistency

- Black stool or dark red blood in the stool (black stools indicates bleeding from the stomach; dark red blood in the stool indicates bleeding from the lower intestine)
- Anemia (could mean that you're bleeding from your gastrointestinal tract)
- Persistent abdominal pain, that is, nothing makes it go away
- New and unusual symptoms, particularly if you're between 45–50 or over 65.
- Weight loss (you've lost at least 5–10 lbs in the last month without trying)

the appropriate tests

You should request the following tests as part of your annual physical:

Visual examination of your rectal area. Here, your doctor looks for visible signs of irritation or inflammation in the rectal area.

Digital rectal exam. In this test the doctor inserts a finger into the rectum to feel for swelling, the condition of your sphincter muscles, and for tenderness, which could be a sign of anal fissures or inflammation. In women, the cervix and a bit of the uterus can be examined, and a condition known as *rectocele* can be checked, where the rectum bulges slightly into the vagina. Anyone engaging in regular anal sex should have this exam annually, too.

Anoscope exam. Here, a short lighted tube similar to, but much shorter than, a sigmoidoscope (see below) is inserted in the rectum to look for signs of inflammation or polyps growth. That said, since a sigmoidoscopy is much more accurate, many specialists recommend you skip the anoscope exam and go directly to sigmoidoscopy.

Occult blood test. Also known as fecal occult blood test (FOBT), this test checks for "hidden" blood in the stools (occult means "hidden"). You collect your own stool samples from three consecutive bowel movements. If blood is found in the stool samples, you'll be referred for a colonoscopy (see below). Certain things in your diet, certain medications, or the presence of hemorrhoids could give you false-positive results. This test detects less than 10 per cent of small polyps, 30–50 per cent of large polyps, and 40–50 per cent of early-stage colorectal cancers. In other words, it may not detect the presence of polyps or cancer.

Sigmoidoscopy. Here a short tube, with a lighted microscope on the end, is inserted about 6 inches into your rectum. The lining of your colon can be examined this way, and any inflammation, polyps (growths which can be benign or malignant), or other abnormalities can be seen. Some doctors use a flexible sigmoidoscope, which is longer (about 2 feet), but since a colonoscope reveals more, there's not much point. This test detects 30–45 per cent of small polyps, and 35–50 per cent of large polyps or early-stage cancers.

Colonoscopy. Prior to this test, you'll need to be cleaned out with laxatives and a liquid diet so the field of vision is clear. Done under sedation, a long fibre-optic lighted tube is inserted into the colon. The tube is about 165 cm long. This enables the doctor to view all sides of the colon, looking for polyps, inflammation, and so on, and allows growths to be removed during the procedure—a particular bonus. A more effective and newer colonoscope is a video colonoscope, which allows a clearer view, in colour, on video. More polyps are found this way than with a fibre-optic colonoscope. This screening tool detects a whopping 85 per cent of small polyps and about 97 per cent of large polyps and early-stage cancers.

Alternate every year between this and sigmoidoscopy.

a word about barium enemas

In light of far more accurate screening tools, such as sigmoidoscopy and colonoscopy, barium enemas are fast becoming the dinosaurs in colon cancer screening. You still need to be cleaned out with laxatives and a liquid diet the night before, but it may be harder to get your bowel movements back to normal after the test because the barium can dry out in the colon and become as hard as concrete. All in all, the black-and-white, two-dimensional images produced by barium X-ray are simply not as accurate as those seen in 3-D colour through colonoscopy or sigmoidoscopy; and you are exposed to a small amount of radiation to boot. Since the test is expensive, and the results may be inconclusive, if not inaccurate—which would warrant colonoscopy anyway—most experts today say, "Skip the barium X-ray and go directly to colonoscopy."

genetic testing for colon cancer

Yes, you can be tested for a colon cancer gene, but the presence of a genetic mutation for colon cancer does not mean you will get colon cancer, nor does the *absence* of a genetic mutation mean that you will not get colon cancer.

Therefore, genetic screening for colon cancer is not meaningful information for most people. Moreover, the stress a positive test can generate may cause more harm than good. If you do test positive for one of the types of colon cancer genes or, more accurately, genetic mutations, you are encouraged to screen more frequently than people who do not have a genetic mutation for colon cancer.

The same ethical dilemmas over genetic testing for breast cancer present themselves when looking at genetic testing for colon cancer. Review chapter 4, pages 103–105 for this discussion.

colon cancer genes

There is one type of colon cancer that does not originate from polyps, known as *hereditary non-polyposis colorectal cancer* (HNPCC). This is a hereditary colorectal cancer that strikes at about age 45. People with this gene may also be at greater risk for cancer of the uterus, bladder or ureter (the orifice out of which we urinate), pancreas, and stomach. Roughly 5 per cent of colorectal cancer is due to an HNPCC gene mutation.

A second gene mutation has been discovered in roughly 6 per cent of the Ashkenazi Jewish population (Jews of Eastern European descent). If you are not Jewish, it is exceedingly rare to test positive for this second kind of mutation.

Finally, less than 1 per cent of colon cancer, known as *familial adenomatous polyposis* (FAP), which is characterized by hundreds of polyps, is linked to a rare genetic mutation.

what to eat

By lowering fat and increasing fibre, you'll greatly reduce your risk of colon cancer, while maintaining good colon health. In fact, experts speculate that by following a low-fat, high-fibre diet, you may be able to avoid 90 per cent of all stomach and colon cancers and 20 per cent of gallbladder, pancreatic, mouth, pharynx, and esophageal cancers. Diet may even play a role in preventing lung cancer; recent studies show that people with low intakes of carotene (orange, red, and purple plant foods), have higher rates of lung cancer.

insoluble fibre

Fibre is the part of a plant your body can't digest, which comes in the form of both water-soluble fibre (dissolves in water) and water-insoluble fibre (does not dissolve in water but instead absorbs water); this is what's meant by "soluble" and "insoluble" fibre. Soluble and insoluble fibre do differ, but they are equally beneficial.

Soluble fibre, discussed in chapter 2, somehow lowers the "bad" cholesterol (LDL) in your body. Insoluble fibre doesn't affect your cholesterol levels at all, but it regulates your bowel movements. How does it do this? As the insoluble fibre moves through your digestive tract, it absorbs water like a sponge and helps to form your waste into a solid form faster, making the stools larger, softer, and easier to pass. Without insoluble fibre, your solid waste just gets pushed down to the colon or lower intestine as always, where it is stored and dried out until you're ready to have a bowel movement.

High-starch foods are associated with drier stools. This condition is exacerbated when you ignore the urge, as the colon will dehydrate the waste even more until it becomes harder and difficult to pass, a condition known as constipation. Insoluble fibre will help to regulate your bowel movements by speeding things along. Insoluble fibre increases the "transit time" by increasing colon motility and limiting the time that dietary toxins hang around the intestinal wall. This is why insoluble fibre can dramatically decrease your risk of colon cancer.

Good sources of insoluble fibre are wheat bran and whole grains, skins from various fruits and vegetables, seeds, leafy greens, and cruciferous vegetables (cauliflower, broccoli, or Brussels sprouts).

what's in a grain?

Most of us turn to grains and cereals to boost our fibre intake, which experts recommend should be at about 25–35 grams per day. Use Table 5.1 to help gauge whether you're getting enough fibre. An easy way to boost your fibre intake is to add pure wheat bran to your foods, which is available in health food stores or supermarkets in a sort of sawdust format. Three tablespoons of wheat bran is equal to 4.4 grams of fibre. Sprinkle 1–2 tablespoons on cereals, rice, pasta, or meat dishes. You can also sprinkle it into orange juice or low-fat yogurt. It has virtually no calories, but it's important to drink a glass of water with your wheat bran, as well a glass of water after you've finished your wheat bran-enriched meal.

TABLE 5.1: FIBRE CONTENT

Cereals (based on 1/2 cup unless otherwise specified)	Grams of fibre
Fibre First	15.0
Fibre One	12.8
All Bran	10.0
Oatmeal (1 cup)	5.0
Raisin Bran (3/4 cup)	4.6
Bran Flakes (1 cup)	4.4
Shreddies (2/3 cup)	2.7
Cheerios (1 cup)	2.2
Corn Flakes (1¼ cup)	0.8
Special K (1¼ cup)	0.4
Rice Krispies (1¼ cup)	0.3
Breads (based on 1 slice)	**Grams of fibre**
Rye	2.0
Pumpernickel	2.0
12-grain	1.7
100 per cent whole wheat	1.3
Raisin	1.0
Cracked-wheat	1.0
White	0

Note: Keep in mind that some of the newer high-fibre breads on the market have up to 7 grams of fibre per slice. This chart is based on what is normally found in typical grocery stores.

fruits and vegetables

Another easy way of boosting fibre content is to know how much fibre your fruits and vegetables pack per serving. All fruits, beans (a.k.a. legumes), and vegetables listed in Table 5.2 show measurements for insoluble fibre, which is not only good for colon health, but for your heart, too. Some of these numbers may surprise you!

TABLE 5.2: FIBRE CONTENT

Fruits	Grams of fibre
Raspberries (3/4 cup)	6.4
Strawberries (1 cup)	4.0
Blackberries (1/2 cup)	3.9
Orange (1)	3.0
Apple (1)	2.0
Pear (1/2 medium)	2.0
Grapefruit (1/2 cup)	1.1
Kiwi (1)	1.0

Beans (based on 1/2 cup unless otherwise specified)	Grams of fibre
Green beans (1 cup)	4.0
White beans	3.6
Kidney beans	3.3
Pinto beans	3.3
Lima beans	3.2

Vegetables (based on 1/2 cup unless otherwise specified)	**Grams of fibre**
Baked potato with skin (1 large)	4.0
Acorn squash	3.8
Peas	3.0
Creamed, canned corn	2.7
Brussels sprouts	2.3
Asparagus (3/4 cup)	2.3
Corn kernels	2.1
Zucchini	1.4
Carrots (cooked)	1.2
Broccoli	1.1

drink water with fibre

How many people do you know who say: "But I *do* eat tons of fibre and I'm still constipated!" Probably quite a few. Well, the reason they remain constipated in spite of their high-fibre diet is that they are not drinking water with fibre. Water means water. Milk, coffee, tea, soft drinks, or juice are not a substitute for water. Unless you drink water with your fibre, the fibre will not bulk up in your colon to create the nice, soft bowel movements you so desire. Think of fibre as a sponge. Obviously, a dry sponge won't work. You must soak it with water in order for it to be useful. Same thing here. *You gotta soak your fibre!* So here is the fibre/water recipe: drink two glasses of water with your fibre. This means having a glass of water with whatever you're eating. Even if what you're eating does not contain much fibre, drinking water with your meal is a good habit to get into. Drink two glasses of water *after* you eat, as well.

There are other reasons to drink lots of water throughout the day. For example, some studies show that dehydration can lead to mood swings and depression. Numerous health and beauty experts often advise women to drink 8–10 glasses of water per day for other reasons: water helps you to lose weight, have well-hydrated, beautiful skin, and urinate regularly, which is important for bladder form and function (women, in particular, can suffer from bladder infections and urinary incontinence). By drinking water with your fibre, you'll be able to get up to that 8–10 glasses of water per day in no time.

vitamins and minerals for the gut

It's believed that fruits and vegetables high in antioxidants, phytoestrogens (plant estrogens, found in soy, discussed in chapter 1), and lignins may also protect against a variety of cancers.

Vitamin A and beta-carotene are associated with preventing or even reversing lung, larynx, colon, prostate, bladder, stomach, esophageal and, possibly, breast cancer.

Vitamins C, E, and selenium are associated with low rates of stomach and esophageal cancers, in particular. It's believed that vitamins C and E block the formation of carcinogenic compounds in the stomach, including polyps.

Vitamin D, which the body naturally makes when exposed to natural light, and calcium have been shown to protect against colorectal and breast cancers. Calcium apparently helps to absorb fecal bile acids, which experts believe promote tumours in the digestive tract.

Epidemiological studies show a higher incidence of colon and breast cancers in regions with less sunlight. (However, this could simply mean that where there's less sunlight, there's more sedentary living.) And finally, epidemiological studies suggest folic acid could lower the risk of colon cancer.

herbs and spices to keep you regular

You may have heard of acidophilus, liquid or powder, as a remedy for chronic constipation, which does not create a dependency.

Or, in Ayervedic medicine, an ancient Indian healing system, triphala is taken to promote regularity and good digestion. Triphala is a combination of three ancient Ayurvedic ingredients: haritaki, bibhitaki, and amalaki. It can be found in most health food stores.

In addition, the following spices are good for digestion, and are not harmful to your colon in any way: licorice root, peppermint leaf, anise seed, yellow dock root, dandelion root, rose petals, coriander seed, celery seed, cinnamon bark, ginger root, cardamom seed, clove bud, and black pepper.

how to move

Following a heart-smart exercise program is good for the gut, too. When oxygen flow is improved throughout your body, everything—including your digestive system—works better. There are also stretches you can do to help strengthen your abdominal muscles, which can help to combat constipation.

1. The Squat. By doing this exercise regularly, you can become more regular, too! Stand with your feet parallel to your hips and slowly squat, making sure your weight is forward (rather than reeling backward, or rolling your knees inward). You may need to practice a few times before you can do this comfortably (see figure i). It's recommended that you squat twice a day to aid with constipation.

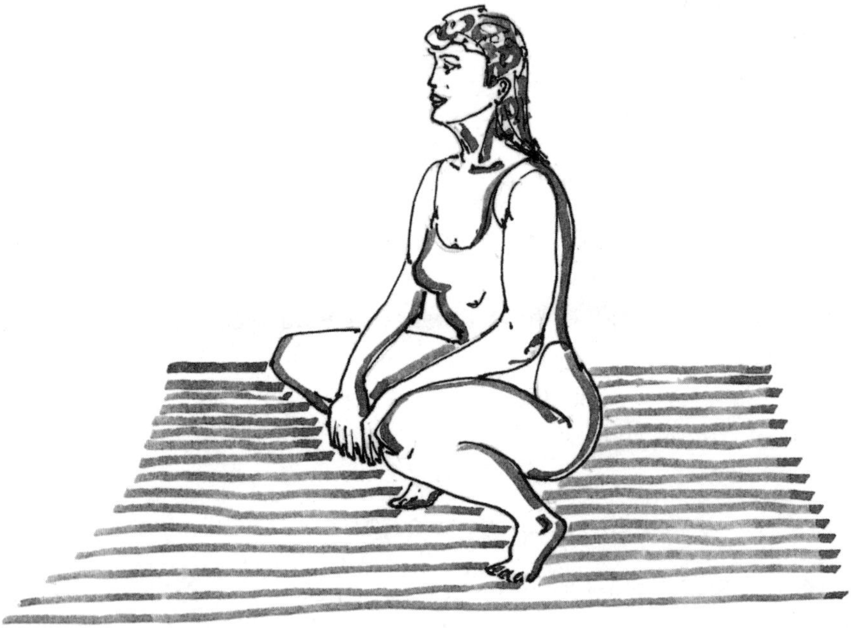

figure i

2. Knee-To-Chest—One Leg. This exercise strengthens your abdominal muscles and, when combined with The Squat (see figure i), can beautifully relieve chronic constipation. Lie on your back on the floor. Bend one knee and bring it in to the chest. Then hug the leg, and slowly bring it toward your abdomen (see figure ii). Hold for a count of 10. Relax and repeat with alternate leg.

3. Knee-To-Chest—Both Legs. This is the same as the one-leg version, only you will bring both legs to the chest and hug them with both arms, bringing them gently toward your abdomen (See Figure iii). Hold for a count of 10. Then relax and repeat.

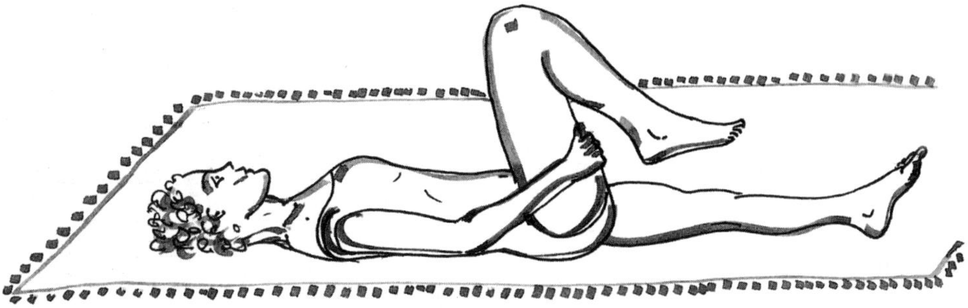

figure ii

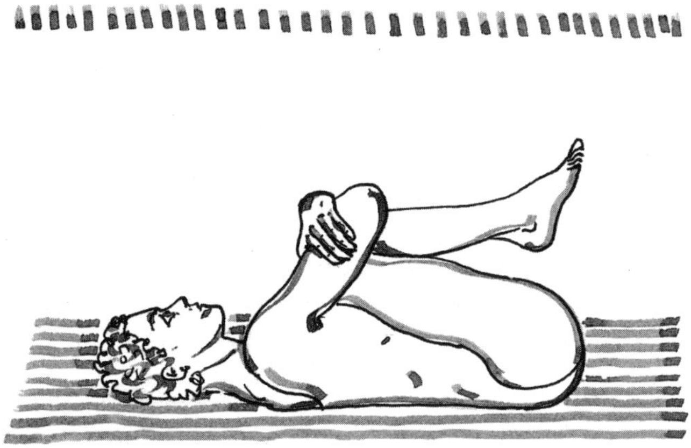

figure iii

six

bone health

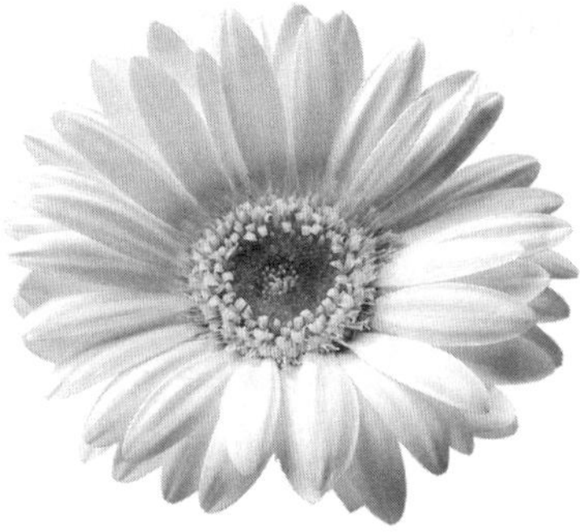

Maintaining bone mass and good bone health is your best defence against bone loss, also known as osteoporosis. Eighty per cent of all osteoporosis sufferers are women, as a direct result of estrogen loss. In Canada, 1.4 million women have osteoporosis; since one in four women over 50 has osteoporosis, that number will climb as women of the '60s begin turning 50.

Although osteoporosis can be disfiguring, it is a relatively silent disease in that there are often no immediate symptoms, pain, or suffering. The problem is not osteoporosis per se, but the risk of fractures. One out of two women over 50 will have an osteoporosis-related fracture in her lifetime. If you have osteoporosis and fall, a fracture can dramatically affect your quality of life. If you've ever experienced reduced mobility, or have had to depend on someone else to prepare meals, shop, or run errands, you have some idea how debilitating being bedridden and immobile can be.

A full 70 per cent of all hip fractures are a direct result of osteoporosis; 20 per cent of those suffering hip fractures will die; 50 per cent will be disabled. In fact, more women die each year as a result of osteoporosis-related fractures than from breast and ovarian cancer combined.

The costs of osteoporosis are taking a toll on our health care system, too. Canada spends $1.3 billion on treating osteoporosis-related fractures each year. The costs are in long-term hospital care and chronic care. By 2025, it's estimated that Canada will need to spend $32.5 billion on treating osteoporosis-related fractures; as your generation ages, the costs will go up.

This chapter explains what osteoporosis is, the dangers of fractures, discusses prevention strategies and therapy. At the end of the chapter, What To Eat offers important information on diet, herbs, and supplements, while How To Move suggests a number of weight-bearing activities that can help you to build bone mass.

what is osteoporosis?

Osteoporosis literally means "porous bones" and is, perhaps, the most feared condition in the postmenopausal community. Unfortunately, osteoporosis is a classic symptom of aging. Normally, by the time a healthy woman reaches her late 30s and 40s, her bones become less dense. By the time she reaches her 50s, she may begin to experience bone loss in her teeth, and become more susceptible to wrist fractures. Gradually, the bones in her spine weaken, fracture, and compress, causing upper-back curvature and loss of height, known as kyphosis, or "dowager's hump." If you've ever been stopped at a traffic light to watch an elderly woman stooped over and struggling to get across the street in time, you've seen osteoporosis in full flare. This does not have to be your fate; there are many ways to maintain bone mass after menopause and prevent the disfiguring effects of bone loss.

why women?

Osteoporosis is more common in women because, typically, when a woman's skeletal growth is completed, she has 15 per cent lower bone mineral density and 30 per cent less bone mass than a man of the same age. Studies also show that women lose more trabecular bone (the inner, spongy part making up the internal support of the bone) at a higher rate than men.

Women are prone to three types of osteoporosis: *postmenopausal, senile*, and *secondary*.

Postmenopausal osteoporosis usually develops roughly 10–15 years after the onset of menopause. In this case, estrogen loss interferes with calcium absorption, and you begin to lose trabecular bone three times faster than the normal rate of trabecular bone loss. You will also begin to lose parts of your cortical bone (the outer shell of the bone) but not as quickly as the trabecular bone. Unlike women, whose estrogen loss dramatically affects bone loss, men never reach a particular age when their testes stop producing testosterone. If they did, they would be just as prone to osteoporosis as women.

Senile osteoporosis affects both men and women. Here, you lose cortical and trabecular bone because of a decrease in bone cell activity that results from aging. Hip fractures are seen most often with this kind of osteoporosis. The decrease in bone cell activity affects your capacity to rebuild bone in the first place, but is also aggravated by low calcium intake.

Secondary osteoporosis means that there is an underlying condition that has caused bone loss. These conditions include: chronic renal (kidney) disease, hypogonadism (an overstimulation of the sex glands, or gonads), hyperthyroidism (an overactive thyroid gland), some forms of cancer, gastrectomy (removal of those parts of the intestine that interfere with calcium absorption), and the use of anticonvulsants.

calcium

Your thyroid gland rents space to cells called C cells, which produce the hormone calcitonin. This hormone helps to regulate calcium and prevent osteoporosis. It is also used to treat Paget's disease, a bone disease which affects mostly men. But to your bones, calcitonin is like a tonsil; it serves a useful purpose, but when the hormone is not manufactured due to the absence of a thyroid gland (if it's removed or ablated because you've been treated for an overactive thyroid gland), you won't really notice any effects, just as you don't miss your tonsils.

Calcium levels are really controlled by the parathyroid glands. Everyone has at least four parathyroid glands that control the body's blood calcium level, or calcium balance. Your parathyroid glands stimulate the release of calcium from the bone to raise blood calcium levels. They also help your body convert vitamin D into calcium.

These glands are located on the back of each lobe of your thyroid gland. The easiest way to grasp exactly where they're located is to imagine the capital letter "H." At each tip of the "H," imagine a circle. If the "H" is your thyroid gland, the circles at each tip are your parathyroid glands.

what causes bone loss anyway?

Our bones are always regenerating, known as remodelling. This process helps to maintain a constant level of calcium in the blood, essential for a healthy heart, blood circulation and blood clotting. About 99 per cent of all the body's calcium is present in the bones and teeth; when blood calcium drops below a certain level, the body will take calcium from the bones to replenish it. By the time we reach our late 30s, our bones lose calcium faster than it can be replaced. The pace of bone calcium loss speeds up for freshly post-menopausal women, who are three to seven years beyond menopause. Bones start absorbing calcium again when this "bone-pause" is past.

The pace then slows once again, but as we age, the body is less able to absorb calcium from food. One of the greatest factors that affects bone loss is estrogen; it slows or even halts the loss of bone mass by improving absorption of calcium from the intestinal tract, which allows us to maintain a higher level of calcium in the blood. The higher the calcium levels in the blood, the less chance of losing calcium from your bones to replenish your calcium blood levels. In men, testosterone does the same thing for them.

There's a long list of other factors that affect bone loss. One of the most obvious is calcium in our diet. Calcium is regularly lost through urine, feces, and dead skin. We need to continuously account for this loss in our diet. In fact, the less calcium we ingest, the more we force our body into taking it out of our bones.

Exercise also greatly affects bone density; the more we exercise, the stronger we make our bones. In fact, the bone mass we have in our late 20s and early 30s will affect our bone mass at menopause.

Finally, there are several physical conditions and external factors that help to weaken our bones, contributing to bone loss later in life. These include:

- Heavy caffeine and alcohol intake. Because they are diuretics, caffeine and alcohol cause you to lose more calcium in your urine. Heavy drinkers tend to suffer from more hip fractures. Since alcohol can damage the liver, which could impair its ability to metabolize vitamin D, it can aggravate bone loss.
- Smoking. Research shows that smokers tend to go into earlier menopause, while older smokers have 20–30 per cent less bone mass than nonsmokers. Several studies show that women who smoke have a greater risk of sustaining fractures than women who do not.

- Women in surgical menopause who are not on ERT. Losing estrogen earlier than you would have naturally increases your bone loss.
- Antacids that contain aluminum and corticosteriods.
- Diseases of the small intestine, liver, and pancreas. These diseases prevent the body from absorbing adequate amounts of calcium from the intestine.
- Lymphoma, leukemia, and multiple myeloma.
- Chronic diarrhea from ulcerative colitis or Crohn's disease (see pages 128–134). This causes calcium loss through feces.
- Surgical removal of part of the stomach or small intestine. This affects absorption.
- Hypercalciuria. In this condition, one loses too much calcium in the urine.
- Early menopause (before age 45). The earlier you stop producing estrogen, the more likely you are to lose calcium (see chapter 1).
- Lighter complexions. Women with darker complexions have roughly 10 per cent more bone mass than fairer women because they produce more calcitonin, the hormone that strengthens bones.
- Low weight. Women with less body fat store less estrogen, which makes the bones less dense to begin with, and more vulnerable to calcium loss.
- Women with eating disorders (yo-yo dieting, starvation diets, binge/purge eaters). When there isn't enough calcium in the bloodstream through diet, the body will go to the bones to get what it needs.
- A family history of osteoporosis. Studies show that women born to mothers with spinal fractures have lower bone mineral density in the spine, neck, and torso.
- High-protein diet. This kind of diet contributes to a loss of calcium in urine.
- Women who have never been pregnant. They haven't experienced the same bursts of estrogen in their bodies as women who have been pregnant.
- Lactose intolerance. Since so much calcium is contained in dairy foods, this allergy is a significant risk factor.
- Teenage pregnancy. When a woman is pregnant in her teens, her bones are not yet fully developed and she can lose as much as 10 per cent of her bone mass unless she has an adequate calcium intake of roughly 2000 mg during the pregnancy and 2200 while breast-feeding.
- Scoliosis, or curvature of the spine.

The most accurate way to measure your risk of osteoporosis is through a bone densitometry, or DEXA, which measures bone mass and provides you with a "fracture risk estimate." This test involves low-dose X-rays and takes about 30 minutes.

thyroid disease and osteoporosis

Women who suffer from an overactive thyroid gland may be at greater risk of bone loss because thyroid hormone will speed up or slow down bone cells just as it will speed up or slow down other functions of the body, such as metabolism.

Osteoblasts are the cells responsible for building bone; osteoclasts are cells that remove old bone so that the new bone can be replaced. When you have an overactive thyroid gland (hyperthyroidism), osteoclasts are overstimulated; in short, they go nuts. They begin to remove bone faster than it can be replaced by the osteoblasts, which are not affected by hyperthyroidism. So you wind up with too much bone removed and bone loss. However, once your hyperthyroidism is treated, and your thyroid hormone replacement medication is balanced, the risk is gone.

If Your Posture Is Affected

Women already affected by bone loss may suffer from slightly curved or disfigured posture, which means that clothing may not hang well. The National Osteoporosis Foundation, in the United States, in partnership with New York's Fashion Institute of Technology, offers the following fashion and design tips:

- Wear clothing that is loose, straight or just slightly fitted
- Wear jeweled, rounded, slight V or soft cowl necklines
- Wear raglan, dropped, or dolman sleeves
- Find pants with elasticized waistbands
- Wear dresses with an empire waist, dropped waist, or A-line
- Make good use of accessories, such as long scarves or shawls to highlight the face and draw eyes up, away from the shoulder area
- Add shoulder pads to compensate for sloping shoulders
- Use backpacks to evenly distribute weight and leave hands free for balance
- Wear flat or low-heeled comfortable slip-on shoes with rubber soles
- Work with department store personal shoppers; their services are usually free

Source: National Osteoporosis Foundation, 1999.

staying hip about fractures

As mentioned at the beginning of this chapter, one in four women over 50 has osteoporosis, and as the '60s generation begins turning 50 in record numbers, we'll be facing a "fractured generation" of sorts—the most debilitating of which are hip fractures. Your risk of a hip fracture is equal to your combined risk of breast, uterine, and ovarian cancer.

In general, all bones are vulnerable to fractures, including the ribs, ankles, and pelvis. Osteoporosis-related fractures are categorized as wrist fractures, vertebral fractures, and the most serious of all, hip fractures, also known as fractures of the proximal femur.

wrist fractures

Wrist fractures start to occur in women who are 50 and older, and the incidence rises until age 65, and then ease off. You break your wrist usually by trying to break a fall. These fractures heal fairly easily and don't lead to serious disability in the same way as hip fractures. However, your wrist will still be stiff or sore, and if you use a computer or work with your hands, the injury will obviously cause discomfort and lost time.

vertebral fractures

These spinal fractures are common within the first 20 postmenopausal years, which means that if your last period was at 53, you can be vulnerable to these fractures until well into your 70s; this is when you could fall on the ice and fracture your tailbone. Women with bone loss in the teeth, or who have already suffered from wrist fractures, which contains trabecular bone, are most at risk for vertebral fractures.

hip fractures

North American women have the highest rates of hip fractures. At 55, you have a 17 per cent chance of sustaining a hip fracture, which compares to only 6 per cent in men of the same age. Women are four times more likely to have a second hip fracture than women without a history of fractures. Most hip fractures occur in Caucasian or Asian women who are in their 70s and 80s. Caucasian women 65 or older have twice the incidence of fractures as women of African descent.

Why are hip fractures so serious? Currently, about 25 per cent of people with hip fractures die from complications, such as pneumonia. The problem begins with being bedridden. You're lying in bed, in pain, on a lot of medication. You just get sicker and sicker until one thing leads to another—actually the fate of many long-term, chronic illness sufferers. In fact, 15–25 per cent are still in long-term care institutions a year after the injury.

Researchers aren't sure whether the high rate of hip fractures in the 70–80-year-olds is due to poor nutrition in younger years. The difference between you and your mother is huge from a nutritional standpoint. Mom grew up during the Depression; you grew up during abundant times, in the 1950s. That said, your mother probably wasn't much of a dieter. Anyone coming of age in the '60s, was exposed to the Twiggy-like thinness which has remained in vogue ever since. And your mother may not have smoked and may not have been as sedentary as you are. So the fracture statistics remain for reasons not currently studied.

eight ways to avoid a fall

If you have suffered some bone loss, here are eight tips to fall-proof your home:

1. Don't leave loose wires, cords, or slippery throw rugs lying around.
2. Make sure you have a nonslip mat in the shower or bathtub.
3. Install night lights to avoid tripping in the middle of the night.
4 Clean up spills on the floors to avoid slipping.
5. Install treads, rails, or rugs (securely) on wooden stairs.
6. Wear comfortable, sturdy shoes with rubber soles.
7. Avoid activity when taking medications that can make you drowsy.
8. Cut down on alcohol consumption: you can fall more easily when you're under the influence of alcohol.

risky movements

If you have more severe bone loss, everyday movements can cause fractures. Watch out for the following: lifting heavy objects (such as groceries) or excessive bending; forceful sneezing or coughing; reaching above your shoulders, as in reaching for something in closets or cupboards; a sudden twist or turn, a movement which you may make when driving; getting in and out of beds or chairs—sitting or lying down in one position for too long can make the normal movements of getting up hazardous. Go slow. To lessen stiffness, which can be quite severe if you have osteoporosis, use a pillow for back support, and avoid cold drafts.

preventing bone loss

There are a few routes you can take to prevent bone loss. The ever-popular diet-and-lifestyle changes is the most natural route, and a route many women feel most comfortable with. Hormone replacement therapy, discussed in chapter 1, is the second route. There are also a few osteoporosis prevention drugs; the most recently approved drug is raloxifene (Evista®), which came to market in 1998, developed by Eli Lilly (see page 156). You cannot combine HRT with Evista®, however. You have to choose. Whichever you choose, you should combine a high-calcium diet and exercise with that therapy.

Neither HRT or Evista® can guarantee freedom from fracture because the bones may still be rigid rather than flexible. Only calcium and exercise can build flexible bone mass. For example, many women who faithfully take estrogen replacement therapy still suffer fractures. That said, when ERT is started at menopause, and continued for the rest of your life, it can reduce the rate of fractures by 40–60 per cent. Women who do not take estrogen, who exercise regularly, and have a diet high in calcium can reduce their rate of fractures by at least 50 per cent, too. However, it's not enough to just take calcium supplements or eat high-calcium foods; you need to cut down on foods that have diuretic qualities: caffeine and alcohol.

How much is enough calcium? According to the National Institutes of Health Consensus Panel on Osteoporosis, premenopausal women require roughly 1000 mg of calcium a day; for perimenopausal or postmenopausal women already on HRT or ERT, 1000 mg, and for peri- and postmenopausal women not taking estrogen, roughly 1500 mg a day. For women who have already been diagnosed with osteoporosis, the Panel recommends 2500 mg of calcium a day.

It's crucial to determine how much calcium you're getting in your diet before you start taking any calcium supplements; too much calcium can cause kidney stones in people who are at risk for them. In addition, not all supplements have been tested for absorbency. In his book *Calcium and Common Sense,* Dr. Robert Heaney suggests that you test absorbency yourself by dropping your supplement into a glass of warm water, then stir occasionally. If the supplement doesn't dissolve completely, chances are it won't be absorbed by your body efficiently.

It's important to remember that a calcium supplement is, in fact, a supplement and should not replace a high-calcium diet. The dosage of your supplement would only need to be roughly 400–600 mg a day, while your diet should account for the remainder of your 1000–1500 daily intake of calcium. Foods that are rich in calcium include all dairy products (an 8 oz glass of milk contains 300 mg calcium), fish, shellfish, oysters, shrimp, sardines, salmon, soybeans, tofu, broccoli, dark green vegetables (except spinach, which contains oxalic acid, a substance that prevents calcium absorption).

osteodoctors

While primary care physicians—family physicians or general practitioners—can manage osteoporosis, if you want to consult a specialist, there are a few you can see, but no, single osteoporosis specialist per se.

Seeing an endocrinologist may be one route, since osteoporosis is a condition associated with estrogen loss and sometimes calcium deficiencies. Rheumatologists, who manage joint pain, are also popular choices, as well as gerontologists, who specialize in aging and diseases of aging. It may be more practical for you to consult a physiotherapist, who can help you strengthen muscles and bones, and even an occupational therapist, who can help you to avoid injuries, get you custom splints or orthopedic equipment to cope with a previous injury. Many people find that visiting an acupuncturist helps to deal with joint pain as well.

osteodrugs

While there are other drugs in development, as of this writing there are four different drug therapies commonly used in preventing and reversing osteoporosis: hormone replacement therapy, selective estrogen receptor modulators, bisphosphorates, and calcitonin. That said, the best prevention therapy, as mentioned above, is a high-calcium diet, combined with exercise. None of the following drug therapies are designed to replace lifestyle changes, and you're encouraged to combine calcium diets and exercise with them.

hormone replacement therapy

By replacing estrogen, you can help to retard the bone-loss process, since it is estrogen that is crucial for calcium absorption in the first place. Not all women should be on estrogen (see chapter 1), while many women do not want to take estrogen, which makes them good candidates for selective estrogen receptor modulators (discussed below). One study shows that postmenopausal women who take two Tums® per day can cut their daily dosage of estrogen in half; half the HRT dose plus two Tums® will prevent bone loss just as well as a full dose of HRT. This is a good option if your reasons for refusing HRT are because of fears of breast cancer risk (see chapter 1). Women in the Tums® study were given two, 600 mg Tums-EXTRA® tablets, a vitamin D supplement to aid calcium absorption by the body, and 0.3 mg of estrogen. The women on low-dosage estrogen showed as much as a 5.2 per cent increase in bone-mass density, which is comparable to higher-dose HRT regimens.

selective estrogen receptor modulators (SERMs)

These are a new class of drugs originally designed to help treat estrogen-dependent breast cancers, but were, instead, shown to help prevent bone loss, particularly around the spine and hip, and even increase bone mass.

The first drug from the SERMs family, approved for use in 1998, is raloxifene (Evista®). Women who took raloxifene for three years reduced their risk of fractures by about 50 per cent. Even better, raloxifene may help protect you from heart disease—good news if you are at risk—because it helps lower "bad" cholesterol (LDL). Some studies suggest that raloxifene may also reduce the incidence of breast cancer in some women—great news for women who cannot take HRT because of a history of breast cancer, for example. Raloxifene and HRT are equally effective in protecting your bones. And, of course, you can continue to take calcium and/or vitamin D with raloxifene.

The bad news is that raloxifene brings with it some estrogen-like side effects, including hot flashes and the risk of blood clots. However, it doesn't cause breast tenderness or bloating. Unlike HRT, raloxifene does not help with the signs of menopause, and may even aggravate them. You cannot take raloxifene unless you are postmenopausal, meaning that you have been free from periods for at least one year. The drug has not been tested in women still having periods. If you are taking warfarin or other coumarin blood thinners, you may also not be a candidate for this drug, and should discuss it with your doctor.

Ideal raloxifene users are postmenopausal women at risk for osteoporosis and heart disease who are not taking HRT, or postmenopausal women at risk for osteoporosis and high risk for breast cancer.

Women who should not take raloxifene include: premenopausal women; pregnant women or women who are breast-feeding; women with a history of blood clots or leg cramps (signs of possible blood clots); women on any form of estrogen or progestin therapy that comes as a pill, patch, or injection; women taking cholestyramine or colestipol; and women with liver problems.

bisphosphonates: bone-forming drugs

As discussed earlier, osteoblasts are the cells responsible for building bone, while osteoclasts are cells that remove old bone so that the new bone can be replaced. Bisphosphonates stop or slow down the osteoclasts, without interfering with osteoblasts, the bone-forming cells. So you wind up with greater bone density. In the past, these drugs were approved only for severe bone diseases, such as Paget's disease. Two bisphosphonates—etidronate (Didrocal/Didronel®) and alendronate (Fosamax®)—have been approved for use in Canada for women who are not on HRT, but who are at risk of osteoporosis. However, bisphosphonates do not relieve any menopausal signs, such as hot flashes, and offers no protection against heart disease.

Bisphosphonates are as effective in reducing the risk of fractures as HRT and raloxifene; the rate is reduced by about 50 per cent in women taking the drug for about three years. If you're taking bisphosphanates, however, you cannot take calcium supplements at the same time, because calcium prevents the body from absorbing the bisphosphonate.

If you're taking alendronate, you'll need to wait 30 minutes after ingesting it before you have food or a calcium supplement. If you're taking etidronate, you'll need to take the drug in a cycle, which your doctor will discuss with you, so you can take calcium supplements. In general, alendronate is a more potent, more effective bisphosphonate. The side effects of etidronate and alendronate may include nausea, abdominal pain or loose bowel movements. In rare instances, some people develop skin rashes or esophageal ulcers.

calcitonin

The hormone calcitonin is sometimes used to slow bone loss in women who are at least five years beyond their menopause; meaning, five years without any periods. However, this is a much cruder way to prevent bone loss, and the hormone can only be taken as an injection or spray because it cannot be metabolized orally. Unlike the drugs discussed above, calcitonin does not help reduce fractures or build bone mass. In fact, calcitonin is fast becoming the dinosaur in osteoporosis prevention, and there are no good reasons to take it in light of the availability of much better therapies.

what to eat

By "boning up" on calcium now, you can fortify yourself against debilitating bone loss. Our bodies lose calcium regulary, and we need to continuously make up for it by ingesting this important nutrient. Remember, to keep your bones healthy, you need 1500 mg of calcuim daily. Calcium can be eaten. And there are many kinds of foods high in calcium. This is your best protection from bone loss, combined with weight bearing activities (see How To Move).

ways to increase calcium intake

Think of calcium as an "RRSP." You want to build up a reserve that your body can use when it ages. Your bones are the "savings account" where all excess calcium is deposited. When the savings account is full, you gain bone mass. When the savings account is depleted, you go into "calcium debt." When this happens, your parathyroid gland produces a hormone that triggers the release of calcium stores from the bone, and you lose bone mass. So in order to keep calcium in that savings account, you have to increase your calcium intake. That means eating three or more calcium-rich foods daily and avoiding foods that cause you to use up or pee out calcium, such as salt, coffee, meat, fluoride, soft drinks, and white-flour products.

maximizing calcium absorption

Calcium is best absorbed in an acidic environment. To increase acidity:

- Drink lemon juice in water with or after your meal.
- Add two tablespoons/30 ml apple cider vinegar and two tablespoons raw honey or blackstrap molasses to a cup/250 ml water; drink with or after your meal.
- Use calcium-rich herbal vinegars in your salad dressing.

calcium greens

Broccoli, kale, turnip greens, or mustard greens contains about 200 mg calcium. One cup cooked collards, wild onions, lamb's quarters, and amaranth greens contain about 400 mg calcium.

The following greens are not high-calcium sources, but high-iron sources: spinach, Swiss chard (silver beet), beet greens, wood sorrel, and rhubarb.

high-calcium sources

Some of these you probably know about; many of these may be new to you:

- Tahini
- Soy or tofu (not all tofu contains calcium; check labels)
- Oats/oatmeal
- Seaweed
- Sardines
- Yogurt
- Nettles
- Dandelion leaves
- Dried fruit (65 mg of calcium is present in 3 small figs, a handful of raisins, 4 dates, or 8 prunes)
- Corn tortillas (because these are made with lime, these are high in calcium)

calcium-rich herbs

A big mug of infusion (see page 33) using any of the following herbs is equal to 250–300 mg of calcium. Add a big pinch of horsetail and increase the calcium content by 10 per cent.

- Nettle
- Sage
- Chickweed
- Red clover
- Comfrey leaf
- Raspberry leaf
- Oatstraw

dairy products

The highest-calcium dairy product is live-culture yogurt, made from milk without hormone and antibiotic residues. Yogurt also strengthens the digestive system, boosts the immune system, eases the nervous system, and helps prevent vaginal infections. Yogurt is much lower in fat than other dairy products, in case you want to stay heart healthy. In fact, 25 per cent (350–400 mg) of your 1500 mg daily calcium requirement can come from 1 cup/250 ml yogurt, which is equal to 1 cup milk, 1 ounce/30 grams hard cheese, or 1/2 cup/115 grams ricotta cheese; 1 cup soy milk yields 80 mg calcium, and 1 cup almond milk yields 165 mg calcium.

calcium supplements

If you can't get enough calcium in your diet, there are always supplements. Calcium supplements are more effective in divided doses. Two doses of 250 mg, taken morning and night, actually provide more usable calcium than a 1000 mg tablet. New research also shows that the amount of calcium absorbed from calcium citrate supplements is consistently higher than the amount absorbed from calcium carbonate supplements.

Popular supplements include: calcium-fortified orange juice, which is easier to digest and absorb then other supplements; calcium citrate in tablet form (crushed tablets are better absorbed); and calcium gluconate, calcium lactate, and calcium carbonate (if chewable). You can take 1500 mg daily of one of these.

A Sample High-Calcium Daily Diet

When making your food choices each day, consider adding some of the following to your menu.

- 1 teaspoon/5 ml seaweed such as kelp
- 2 cups/500 ml fresh or 1 cup/250 ml cooked dark greens
- 1 cup yogurt or whey
- a big mug of calcium-rich herbal infusion
- 1 tablespoon herbal vinegar
- 1 tablespoon lemon juice in which eggshell has soaked overnight
- 2 tablespoons blackstrap molasses

other bone supplements

The following are also high in nutrients that will promote bone health.

- Fruits and vegetables high in zinc, magnesium, potassium (slows calcium excretion), fibre, and vitamin C (aids in bone formation), can keep bones strong and fracture free.
- Wild yam cream, which also contains a naturally derived progesterone.
- Supplements of up to 50,000 units beta-carotene daily. Increases progesterone production and protects bones.
- Microcrystalline hydroxapatite. Specifically formulated to deposit minerals into the bones. Helps reverse osteoporosis and heal compression fractures in the spine.

- Vitamin D supplements (if you cannot spend 10–15 minutes in the sun daily). Recommended dose is 400–800 IU daily.
- Horsetail herb (*Equisetum arvense*). Increases calcium absorption.
- Dandelion root tincture. Increases calcium absorption.

how to move

As one fitness expert told me: "If you want a strong house, you need a strong frame." When you increase the load on your bones, your bones increase in mass; similarly, when you decrease the load on your bones, they decrease in mass. And the denser your bones, the harder they are to break or sprain. To combat osteoporosis, therefore, exercises that build bone mass are important.

weight-bearing and resistance exercise

Carrying weights is one of the best ways to increase bone mass, while doing weight-bearing activities also builds bone mass and uses up calories. By increasing muscular strength through these activities, we also increase flexibility (to help combat falls) and endurance. For example, you'll find that the first time you ride your bike from home to downtown, your legs may feel sore. Do that same ride 10 times, and your legs will no longer feel sore. That's what's meant by building endurance. Of course, you won't be as out of breath, either, which is another way of building endurance.

Hand weights or resistance exercises (using rubber-band products or pushing certain body parts together) help increase lean body mass—body tissue that is not fat. That is why many people find their weight does not drop when they begin to exercise. Leg lifts and arm lifts with weights increase balance, bone strength, and help maintain flexibility. Begin with 1-pound weights and increase slowly to 4–5 pounds.

Other forms of resistance exercise involve moving objects or your own body weight to create resistance, using equipment at your gym or fitness centre or even common household objects such as water jugs or canned goods. Attaching Velcro weights to your wrists and ankles and just moving around as you normally would is also a good way to increase resistance.

As your muscles become bigger, and your bones become denser, your body fat decreases. It's recommended that you do weight-bearing exercise four times a week for 30 minutes.

enjoyable activities that help build bone mass

Try to choose one activity from this list that is your enjoyable sport. If you enjoy your activity, you'll do it more often.

- Walking
- Jogging
- Hiking
- Cross-country skiing
- Weightlifting
- Climbing stairs
- Bowling
- Dancing
- Badminton
- Volleyball
- Running
- Bicycling
- Tai chi
- Gardening
- Snowshoeing
- Tennis
- Rowing
- Water workouts
- Basketball
- Soccer

seven

type 2 diabetes

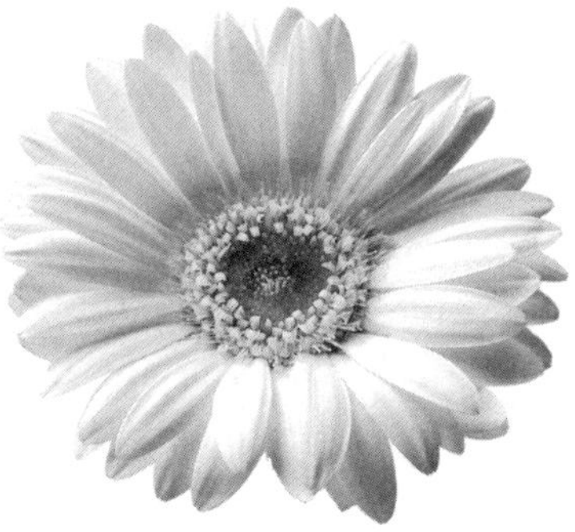

By 2004, one in four North Americans over the age of 45 will be diagnosed with Type 2 diabetes; 65–70 per cent of those diagnosed with Type 2 diabetes are women, while according to some experts, about 95 per cent of women with Type 2 diabetes are obese. Women are more prone to Type 2 diabetes because they have more body fat than men. Women require more weight to protect their reproductive organs; women also tend to gain weight during pregnancy and after childbirth, and will lose 25 per cent of their metabolic efficiency after menopause. If you were diagnosed with Type 2 diabetes before menopause, issues such as fluctuating blood sugar levels, heart disease, osteoporosis, and even breast cancer risk can factor into your diabetes management decisions after menopause.

what is type 2 diabetes?

Diabetes wasn't officially labelled Type 1 and Type 2 until 1979. Type 2 diabetes means that your pancreas is functioning. You are making plenty of insulin. In fact, you are probably making too much insulin, a condition called *hyperinsulinemia*. Insulin is a hormone made by your beta cells, the insulin-producing cells within the islets of Langerhans—small islands of cells afloat in your pancreas. The pancreas is a bird beak-shaped gland situated behind the stomach.

Insulin is a major player in our bodies. One of its most important functions is to regulate blood sugar levels. It does this by acting as a sort of courier, knocking on your cells' door, and announcing: "Sugar's here; come and get it!" Your cells then open the door to let sugar in from your bloodstream. That sugar is absolutely vital to your health, and provides you with the energy you need to function.

What happens if the cells don't answer the door? Two things. First, the sugar in your bloodstream will accumulate, having nowhere to go, analogous to the kind of situation that develops when your newspapers pile up outside the door when you're away. Second, your pancreas will keep sending out more couriers to try to get your cells to open that door and take in the "newspapers." The result of the cells' not complying is a pile of newspapers *and* a line-up of unsuccessful couriers by your door.

When the cell doesn't answer the door, this is called *insulin resistance*; the cell is resisting insulin. The end result, however, is *diabetes*, which means "high blood sugar." A synonym for diabetes is *hyperglycemia,* which also means "high blood sugar." If insulin resistance goes on for too long, the pancreas can become overworked and eventually may not make enough, or any, insulin. In effect, it's like a courier strike. And finally, the liver, being the good neighbour that it is, will lend a bowl or two of sugar to the sugar-deprived cell. But this can exacerbate existing high blood sugar.

Type 2 diabetes, a genetic disease, is a completely different disease than Type 1 diabetes, an autoimmune disease, also known as juvenile diabetes or insulin-dependent diabetes mellitus (IDDM). Only 10 per cent of all people with diabetes have Type 1 diabetes. Type 2 diabetes, on the other hand, accounts for 90 per cent of all people with diabetes. Since Type 2 diabetes doesn't usually develop until after age 45, it was once known as *mature-onset diabetes* or *adult-onset diabetes*. And since Type 2 diabetes is a disease of insulin resistance, rather than no insulin, it often can be managed through diet and exercise, without insulin injections. For this reason, Type 2 diabetes was also known as *non-insulin-dependent diabetes mellitus* (NIDDM). All of these labels have been replaced by "Type 2 diabetes."

Here's where it gets *really* confusing! When you are told that you have non-insulin-dependent diabetes, it doesn't mean that some day you *won't* require insulin. Insulin resistance, characterized by the body's inability to use insulin, sometimes leads to a condition in which the pancreas stops making insulin altogether. The cells' resistance to insulin makes the pancreas work harder, causing too much insulin in the system (*hyperinsulinemia*) until it stops producing insulin. Your pancreas is making the insulin and knocking on the door, but the cells aren't answering. Your pancreas will eventually say, "Okay, fine! I'll shut down production since you obviously aren't using what I'm making." A lot of people with Type 2 diabetes will therefore confuse *requiring* insulin with Type 1 diabetes, falsely believing that their Type 2 diabetes has turned into Type 1. Type 2 diabetes cannot "turn into" Type 1 diabetes any more than an apple can turn into a banana. So what do you call it when someone with Type 2 diabetes requires insulin? Try *insulin-requiring Type 2 diabetes*. In fact, about one-third of all people with Type 2 diabetes will eventually need to begin insulin therapy.

Something else you need to understand about Type 2 diabetes is that the high blood sugar that results from insulin resistance can lead to a number of other diseases, including cardiovascular disease (heart disease and stroke) and peripheral vascular disease (PVD), which means that the blood doesn't flow properly to other parts of your body. This can create a number of problems; many people who suffer a heart attack or stroke have Type 2 diabetes.

who's at risk?

If you consume a diet higher in fat than carbohydrates, and low in fibre, you increase your risk for Type 2 diabetes if you are genetically predisposed to the disease. If you weigh at least 20 per cent more than you should for your height and age (the technical definition of "obese"—see chapter 3), are sedentary, and over age 45, you are considered at high risk for Type 2 diabetes. Seventy-three per cent of all women with diabetes are obese.

Your risk further increases if you have high cholesterol or high blood pressure; smoke; are of aboriginal descent (this is true for aboriginal peoples all over the world, from Australia to North America; in Canada, First Nations people are at highest risk; in the United States, the Pima Indians are at highest risk); are of African or Hispanic descent; have a family history of Type 2 diabetes; or have a history of gestational diabetes.

impaired glucose tolerance (IGT)

Prior to September 1998, many people with Type 2 diabetes were told they had *impaired glucose tolerance* (IGT), which has also been called "borderline diabetes."

For the record, there is no such thing as borderline diabetes. And in light of new guidelines, there is no longer any such thing as impaired glucose tolerance, either. But here's what it meant before September 1998: IGT was what many doctors referred to as the "gray zone" between normal blood sugar levels and "full-blown diabetes." Normal fasting blood sugar levels (what they are before you've eaten) are between 3–5 millimoles (mmol), a unit of measurement that counts molecular volume per litre. In the past, three fasting blood glucose levels between 5–7.8 mmol meant that you had IGT. A fasting blood glucose level over 7.8 mmol or a random (any time of day) blood glucose level greater than 11.1 mmol meant that you had diabetes.

That's all changed. Today, anyone with a fasting blood sugar level higher than 7 mmol/L is considered to be in the diabetic range, and is officially diagnosed with Type 2 diabetes.

signs and symptoms

If you have any of the symptoms listed below, request to be screened for Type 2 diabetes, which can be done through a simple blood test:

- Weight gain. When you're not using your insulin properly, you may suffer from excess insulin, which can increase your appetite. This is a classic Type 2 symptom.
- Blurred vision or any change in sight (often there is a feeling that your prescription eyewear is weak).
- Drowsiness or extreme fatigue at times when you shouldn't be drowsy or tired.
- Frequent infections that are slow to heal. Be on the alert for recurring vaginal yeast infections or vaginitis, which means vaginal inflammation, characterized by itching and/or foul-smelling discharge.
- Tingling or numbness in the hands and feet.
- Gum disease. High blood sugar affects the blood vessels in your mouth, causing inflamed gums; the sugar content can get into your saliva, causing cavities in your teeth.

Diabetes experts point out that the following may also be signs of Type 2 diabetes:

- Irregular menstrual periods, such as changes in cycle length or flow (this could be a sign of menopause as well, discussed in chapter 1)
- Depression, which could be a symptom of either low or high blood sugar (see chapter 8)
- Headaches (from hypoglycemia)
- Insomnia and/or nightmares (from hypoglycemia)
- Spots on the shin (known as *necrobiosis diabeticorum*)
- Decaying toenails
- Muscle pains or aches after exercise (high blood sugar can cause lactic acid to build up, which can cause pain that prevents you from continuing exercise)

You may also have diabetes if your doctor has diagnosed you with the following: high cholesterol; high blood pressure; anemia; cataracts; salivary-gland stones

controlling your blood sugar

Controlling your blood sugar means testing your blood sugar, meal planning (see What To Eat), and exercising (see How To Move). By controlling your blood sugar, you will stay free of the symptoms of diabetes as well as reduce your risks of complications.

blood sugar testing

The equipment you need for self-testing blood sugar is a good glucose meter. There are several on the market; your doctor, pharmacist, or diabetes educator can recommend the right brand for you. When you get your glucose meter, experts suggest you compare your results to one regular laboratory test, to make sure you've purchased a reliable and accurate machine.

Today, most glucose meters measure glucose levels in plasma. What this means is that if you're a self-testing veteran, your next glucose meter may suddenly be giving you readings that are 12 per cent higher than your last meter. This doesn't mean that you are losing control of your disease; rather, it means that your meter is measuring glucose levels in your plasma instead of whole blood. As a rule, before you purchase a new glucose meter, make sure you ask the pharmacist: "Is this a whole blood test or a plasma test?" Moreover, discuss with your health care practitioner how frequently to test yourself as a general guideline for testing times (see pages 169–170).

choosing and using your glucose meter

All glucose meters will provide the following: a battery-powered, pocket-sized device; an LED screen (that is, a calculator-like screen); accurate results in 30 to 60 seconds; the date and time of your test result; a recall memory of at least your last 10 readings; at least a one-year warranty; the opportunity to upgrade; a 1-800 customer service hotline; mailings and giveaways every so often; and a few free lancets with your purchase; you may have to purchase separately a lancing device, a sort of Pez dispenser for your lancets. (Eventually, you'll run out of lancets and have to buy those, too.)

No matter which glucose meter you choose, use these instructions to guide you through the self-testing process:

- Wash your hands with an antibacterial soap.
- Pierce your finger on the side rather than top, and obtain a "hanging" drop of blood (some newer devices "suck out" your blood for you).
- Smear or blot your drop of blood onto a plastic strip that looks like a strip of tape without the sticky side. (Whether you smear or wipe depends on your glucose meter.)
- Turn on your glucose meter and place the strip into the machine.
- The results will show up on the calculator-like screen.
- Record these results in a logbook. A good result before meals ranges from 4–7 mmol/L; a good result after meals ranges from 5–10 mmol/L.

factors that can taint your results

Most people are not testing their blood sugar under squeaky-clean laboratory conditions. The following outside factors may interfere with your meter's performance.

- *Other medications you're taking.* Studies show that some meters can be inaccurate if you're taking acetaminophen, salicylate, ascorbic acid, dopamine, or levodopa. As a rule, if you're taking any medications, check with your doctor, pharmacist, and glucose meter manufacturer (call manufacturer's 1-800 number) about whether your medications can affect the meter's accuracy.

- *Humidity*. The worst place to keep your meter and strips is in the bathroom, where humidity can ruin your strips, unless they're individually wrapped in foil. Keep your strips in a sealed container away from extreme temperatures. Use your "video" rules; don't store your meter and strips in a hot glove compartment, for example. Don't keep them in the freezer, either.
- *Bright light*. Ever tried to use a calculator or portable computer in bright sunlight? It's not possible because the light interferes with the screen. Some meters are photometric, which means they are affected by bright light. If you plan to test in sunlight, get a biosenser meter that is unaffected by bright light (there are several).
- *Touching the test strip*. Many glucose meters come with test strips that cannot be touched with your fingers or a second drop of blood. If you're all thumbs, purchase a meter that is unaffected by touch and/or allows a second drop of blood.
- *Wet hands*. Before you test, thoroughly dry your hands. Water can dilute your blood sample.
- *Motion*. It's always best to test yourself when you're standing still. Testing on planes, trains, automobiles, buses, and subways may affect your results, depending on the brand of glucose meter.
- *Dirt, lint, and blood*. Particles of dirt, lint, and old blood can sometimes affect the accuracy of a meter, depending on the brand. Make sure you clean the meter regularly (follow the manufacturer's cleaning directions) to remove buildup. Make sure you change your batteries, too! There are meters on the market that do not require cleaning and are unaffected by dirt, but they may cost a little more.

when to test your blood sugar

It makes the most sense to test yourself before each meal, so you know what your levels are before you eat anything, as well as about two hours after meals.

Immediately after eating, everybody's blood sugar is high, so this is not the ideal time to test levels. In a person without diabetes, blood sugar levels will drop about two hours after eating, in response to the natural insulin the body makes. Similarly, test yourself two hours after eating to make sure that you are able to "mimic" a normal blood sugar pattern, too. Ideally, this translates into at least four blood tests daily: when you wake up; after breakfast/before lunch (two hours after breakfast); after lunch/before dinner (two hours after lunch); after dinner or at bedtime (two hours after dinner).

The most revealing information about your blood sugar control is in the answers to the following questions:

1. What is your blood sugar level as soon as you wake up? (It should be at its lowest point.)
2. What is your blood sugar level two hours after a meal? (It should be much lower two hours after eating than one hour after eating.)
3. What is your blood sugar level when you feel ill? (You need to avoid dipping too low or high, since your routine is changing.)

glycosylated hemoglobin

The most detailed blood sugar test cannot be done at home yet. This is a blood test that checks for glycosylated hemoglobin (glucose attached to the protein in your red blood cells), known as *glycohemoglobin* or HbA1c levels. This test can tell you how well your blood sugar has been controlled over a period of two to three months by showing what percentage of it is too high. This test is comparable to the gas-tank meters in cars that can tell you what percentage of your last quarter tank is left before you need to refuel. That information is far more telling than just "F," "1/2," "1/4," and "E." It's recommended that see your doctor for an HbA1c test every 3 months.

managing low blood sugar

When you're diagnosed with Type 2 diabetes, whether your treatment revolves around lifestyle modification, oral hypoglycemic or insulin therapy, you may experience an episode of low blood sugar, clinically known as hypoglycemia. Hypoglycemia can sometimes come on suddenly, particularly overnight. If left untreated, it can also result in coma, brain damage, and death. In the past, hypoglycemia was a more common problem among people with Type 1 diabetes. But since 40–50 per cent of all people with Type 2 diabetes will eventually graduate to insulin therapy, the incidence of hypoglycemia has increased by 300 per cent in this group. Moreover, hypoglycemia is a common side effect of oral hypoglycemic pills (see pages 171–173) , the medication the majority of Type 2 suffers take when they are first diagnosed. Note that any blood sugar reading below 3.8 mmol/L is considered too low.

medications and insulin

There are four kinds of medications that may be prescribed to you when diet and lifestyle changes make no impact on your blood sugar levels. It's crucial to note, however, that these medications can only be prescribed to people who still produce insulin. They have no effect on those with Type 1 diabetes, or insulin-dependent diabetes. Before you fill your prescription for anti-diabetic pills, you should know that between 40–50 per cent of all people with Type 2 diabetes require insulin therapy after 10 years. Continuing insulin resistance may cause you to stop responding to oral medications. It is also important to note that these pills are meant to complement your meal plan, exercise routine, and glucose monitoring; they are not a substitute.

Bear in mind, too, that physicians who prescribe anti-diabetic medications are not helping you manage your diabetes properly if they are not working with you to modify your diet and lifestyle. These medications should be prescribed only after you've been unsuccessful in managing your Type 2 diabetes through lifestyle modification and frequent blood sugar testing.

If you cannot get down to a healthy body weight, you are probably a good candidate for anti-diabetic medication. And people with Type 2 diabetes who cannot control their blood sugar levels despite lifestyle changes are also good candidates for the medications discussed below.

oral hypoglycemic agents (OHAs)

Sulphonylureas and biguanides are common oral hypoglycemic agents (OHAs). Sulphonylureas are pills that help your pancreas release more insulin; biguanides help your insulin work better. Initially, 75 per cent of people with Type 2 diabetes will respond well to sulphonylureas, while biguanides will lower blood sugar in 80 per cent of people with Type 2 diabetes. About 15 per cent of all people treated with OHAs fail to respond to them at all, while 3–5 per cent of all people on OHAs will stop responding to them each year. So don't get too comfortable on these pills.

Sulphonylureas would generally be the initial oral agent of choice in people who are not obese and/or have high blood sugar levels, or suffer from symptoms of high blood sugar. A biguanide is appropriate in people who *are* obese and have milder levels of high blood sugar. That's because biguanides do not result in the weight gain that is typically associated with sulphonylureas and insulin therapy.

dosages for sulphonylureas

There is no fixed dosage for sulphonylureas. It all depends on the brand of pill. For example, it's common to take anything from 80–320 mg a day. If you are taking a dosage higher than the recommended initial dose, you should divide your dose into two equal parts. Pills should be taken before or with meals, and your doctor should start you on the lowest effective dose. If your blood sugar levels are high when you start your pills, it's a good idea to have a short trial period of about six to eight weeks to make sure the drug is working.

dosages for biguanides (Metformin)

There is only one biguanide available in Canada, which goes by the name Metformin. In this case, the usual dose is 500 mg three or four times a day, or 850 mg two or three times a day. Your dose is not to exceed 2.5 grams a day. If you're elderly, your doctor will probably prescribe a lower dose.

when OHAs should not be used

If you've had Type 2 diabetes longer than 10 years, this is not the time to start OHAs. And, of course, nobody with Type 1 or insulin-dependent diabetes should ever take OHAs; they will not work. OHAs should never be taken under the following conditions, either: alcoholism; pregnancy; kidney or liver failure (Metformin only).

side effects

Sixty per cent of people taking OHAs continue to have high blood sugar levels two hours after meals. OHAs can also cause increased appetite and weight gain. However, the main side effect with OHAs is hypoglycemia (low blood sugar), which occurs in one in five people treated with OHAs. If you're over age 60, hypoglycemia may occur more often, which is why it's dangerous for anyone over age 70 to take certain OHAs.

About one-third of all people taking OHAs will experience gastrointestinal side effects; no appetite, nausea, abdominal discomfort and, with Metformin, diarrhea.

Adjusting dosages and taking your pills with your meals or afterward often clears up the above symptoms.

acarbose (a.k.a. alpha-glucosidase inhibitors)

Acarbose is a pill that delays the breakdown of sugar in your meal by delaying the conversion of starch and sucrose into glucose; this reduces high blood sugar levels after you eat. Acarbose is prescribed to people who cannot seem to get their postmeal or postprandial (after-meal) blood sugar levels down to acceptable levels.

A major benefit of acarbose is that it may reduce the risk of hypoglycemic episodes during the night, particularly in insulin users. Researchers are studying the possible use of acarbose as a substitute for that "morning insulin."

In terms of dosage, the usual rules apply: acarbose should complement your meal plan and exercise routine; it is not a substitute or way out, and does not, by itself, cause hypoglycemia.

thiazoladinediones (troglitazone or Rezulin™)

These pills make your cells more sensitive to insulin, thereby improving insulin resistance. When this happens, more glucose gets into your tissues, and less glucose hangs around in your blood. The result is that you'll have lower fasting blood glucose levels, without the need to increase insulin levels.

Troglitazone works by stimulating muscle tissue to drink in glucose. It also decreases glucose production from the liver, and makes fat tissue more receptive to glucose. This drug is reserved for people with Type 2 diabetes who must take insulin to reduce their blood sugar levels.

when you need to take insulin

Forty to 50 per cent of all people with Type 2 diabetes require insulin injections to manage their condition. Many doctors often delay prescribing insulin therapy for as long as possible by prescribing maximum doses of the anti-diabetic pills discussed above. This approach isn't considered good diabetes management. If you need insulin, you should take insulin. The goal is to get your disease under control.

Anyone with the following conditions is a candidate for insulin therapy: high blood sugar levels, despite maximum doses of OHAs; fasting glucose levels consistently over 9 mmol/L; illness or stress (insulin may be needed until you recover); complications of diabetes; pregnancy (insulin therapy may be temporary).

If going on insulin will affect your job security, discuss this with your doctor so that appropriate documents can be drafted to your employer. Also keep in mind that if insulin therapy does not bring your diabetes under control within six months, it may be necessary to return to your drug therapy. And, let me dispel a common fear about insulin: since insulin is not a blood product, you don't have to worry about being infected with a blood-borne virus such as HIV or hepatitis.

the right insulin

The goal of a good insulin program is to try to mimic what your pancreas would do if it were working properly. Blood sugar rises in a sort of "wave" pattern. The big waves come in after a big meal; the small waves come in after a small meal or snack. The insulin program that is prescribed for you needs to be matched to your own particular wave pattern. So what you eat—and when—has a lot to do with the right insulin program. Therefore, the right insulin for someone who eats three square meals a day may not be appropriate for someone who tends to graze all day. And the right insulin for an active 47-year-old man in a stressful job may not be the right insulin for a 67-year-old woman who does not work, and whose heart condition prevents her from exercising regularly.

You and your health care team must also decide how much control you need over your blood sugar. Insulin "recipes" depend on whether you need tight control (3–6 mmol), medium control (4–10 mmol), and even loose control (11–13 mmol). Loose control is certainly not encouraged, but on rare occasions—for example, when a person is elderly and suffering from a number of other health problem—it is still done.

To determine the appropriate insulin recipe for you, your health care team should look at who you are as a person—what you eat, where you work (do you work shifts?), your willingness to change your eating habits, and other lifestyle factors.

concerns for women with type 2 diabetes

In a survey of the general Canadian population, 11 per cent of those between 65 and 74 reported having diabetes. Since heart disease is a major complication of Type 2 diabetes, and women are more prone to heart disease as a result of estrogen loss after menopause, the recommendation is that women with Type 2 diabetes seriously consider hormone replacement therapy after menopause. The Women's Health Initiative (WHI) is currently studying 25,000 postmenopausal women, many of whom have diabetes. The results of this study, anticipated by 2003, are expected to present more concrete facts regarding the perceived benefits of HRT on postmenopausal women with Type 2 diabetes.

Many women with Type 2 diabetes, who are on HRT, will also be concerned about their risk of breast cancer. Taking estrogen can stimulate or trigger the growth of an estrogen-dependent breast cancer cell (a breast cancer cell that "feeds" or thrives on the hormone estrogen). Taking the osteoporosis prevention drug raloxifene (see chapter 6) may be an alternative, since raloxifene has been shown to protect against heart disease, and may even lower the incidence of breast cancer in some women. And since many more women die of a heart attack than breast cancer, particularly if they have Type 2 diabetes, the thought of preventing heart disease, as well as fractures from osteoporosis is considered to be a benefit.

In postmenopausal women with diabetes, the risk of heart disease is two to three times higher than in the general female population. Furthermore, as estrogen and progesterone levels drop, women with diabetes can expect fluctuations in their blood sugar levels, and possibly more episodes of low blood sugar. After menopause, women taking insulin may find that their insulin requirements have dropped by 20 per cent, too.

menopause and blood sugar

As you approach menopause, you'll want to revisit your blood sugar monitoring habits. That's because menopause often masks the symptoms of low or high blood sugar, and vice versa. For example, hot flashes, moodiness, and short-term memory loss are also associated with low blood sugar. Experts recommend that before you decide that you're low and bite into that chocolate bar, you should test your blood sugar first to determine if your symptoms are caused by sugar or hormones. Otherwise, ingesting more sugar than you need could cause high blood sugar unnecessarily.

That said, many women find that because their estrogen and progesterone levels are dropping, they experience more frequent and severe episodes of low blood sugar. As mentioned earlier, estrogen can trigger insulin resistance; the loss of estrogen will therefore have the opposite effect, causing insulin to be taken up more quickly by the body, which could result in low blood sugar. An easy way to remember how estrogen levels affect blood sugar is to note that when estrogen is up, so is blood sugar; when estrogen is down, so is blood sugar. Therefore, high estrogen levels equals high blood sugar; low estrogen levels equals low blood sugar.

The only way to cope with these fluctuations is to try to eliminate other causes for blood sugar fluctuations, such as stress, deviating from meal and exercise plans, and so on. If you're on OHAs, you may need to adjust your dosages around menopause to compensate for less resistance to insulin as your hormone levels drop. If you go on hormone replacement therapy, you may need to readjust your dosages again.

If you have persistent high blood sugar levels, you may find the normal menopausal symptoms, such as vaginal dryness, for example, exacerbated. In this case, if you gain more control over blood sugar levels, your menopausal symptoms may be less severe.

mood swings

Mood swings can be an especially tricky symptom of both menopause and fluctuating blood sugar levels. Many women with diabetes struggle with severe mood swings, which can make controlling blood sugar more difficult. While anger and depression can be symptoms of low blood sugar, anxiety and irritability can be symptoms of high blood sugar. Factor in hormonal changes during menopause, and moods can be severely affected.

Unfortunately, depression and irritability can lead women to poor diabetes control. Frequent monitoring of your blood sugar levels and sticking to your meal plan can help to prevent drastic mood swings. (For more about mood swings, see chapter 8.)

what to eat

By following the guidelines in What To Eat for chapters 2 and 3, you'll be well on your way to managing Type 2 diabetes. A diet high in fibre (see chapter 5) will slow down the rate at which your food breaks down into glucose, a process known as delayed glucose absorption. In addition, you should also learn about meal planning and follow the Canadian Diabetes Association meal planning guidelines, outlined here.

meal plans

Meal plans recommended by registered dietitians are tailored to your individual goals and medication regimen. Men and women will usually require different quantities of food. The goal is to keep the supply of glucose consistent by spacing out your meals, snacks, and activity levels accordingly. If you lose weight, this will allow your body to use insulin more effectively, but not all people with Type 2 diabetes need to lose weight. If you're on insulin, meals will have to be timed to match your insulin's peak. A dietitian can be helpful by customizing a meal plan that addresses your specific needs (weight control, shiftwork, travel, and so on).

A good meal plan will ensure that you are getting enough nutrients to meet your energy needs, and that your food is spread out over the course of the day. For example, if your meal plan allots three meals, with one to two snacks, meals should be spaced four to six hours apart so your body isn't overwhelmed. If you are obese, snacks will likely be discouraged because they can both cause you to oversecrete insulin and increase your appetite. A meal plan should also help you to eat consistently rather than bingeing one day and starving the next.

A good meal plan will also ensure that you're getting the vitamins and minerals you need without taking supplements, such as iron, calcium, folic acid, vitamins A, B_1, B_2, B_3, C, D, and E.

Golden Rules of Diabetes Meal Plans

1. Eat three meals a day at fairly regular times, spaced four to six hours apart.
2. Ask your dietitian to help you plan your snacks.
3. Try to eat a variety of foods each day from all food groups—fruits and vegetables, meat and alternatives, grain products, and dairy products.
4. Learn how to gauge serving sizes; volume of bowls and glasses, and so on.
5. Ask your dietitian or diabetes educator about how to adjust your diet if you're travelling (this depends on whether you're on medication, where you're going, what foods will be available, and so on.)
6. Draw up a Sick Days Plan with your dietitian. This regimen will depend on what your regular meal plan includes.
7. Ask about any meal supplements, such as breakfast bars, sports bars, or meal replacement drinks. How will these figure into your meal plan?
8. Choose lower-fat foods more often.
9. Before you shop for food, learn the Food Choice Values and Symbols system. Developed by the Canadian Diabetes Association (CDA), it will tell you how various foods can be incorporated into your meal plan. This system is different from the Food Exchange lists developed by the American Diabetes Association (ADA). The CDA has created seven symbols (colour- and shape-coded) to represent various food groups. There are many crossovers, however; many of these food categories are a combination of carbohydrates, sugar, or fat.

delayed glucose absorption

Guar gum is a high source of fibre made from the seeds of the Indian cluster bean. When you mix guar with water, it turns into a gummy gel, which slows down your digestive system, similar in effect to acarbose (see pages 172–173).

Guar has often been used as a natural substance to treat high blood sugar as well as high cholesterol. Guar can cause gas, some stomach ache, nausea, and diarrhea. (These are also side effects of acarbose.) The problem with guar is that, to date, there are no scientific studies concluding that it improves blood sugar control. Nevertheless, most experts agree that it can certainly provide some marginal benefits.

Delay glucose absorption by eating more fibre, avoiding table sugar (sucrose), and eating smaller meals more often to space out your calories.

how to move

More than 50 per cent of all people with diabetes exercise less than once a week, and 56 per cent of all diabetes-related deaths are due to heart attacks. By following the guidelines under How To Move in chapters 2, 3, and 6, you'll be doing all the right moves for managing Type 2 diabetes, too. Exercise can be tremendously beneficial and life-extending. If you've been sedentary most of your life, there's nothing wrong with starting off with simple, even leisurely activities. Just get moving!

sugar and muscles

When you think "muscle," think "sugar." Every time you work any muscle in your body, either independent of an aerobic activity, or during an aerobic activity, your muscles use up glucose from your bloodstream as fuel.

Forty per cent of your body weight is made from muscle, where sugar is stored. The muscles use this sugar when they are being worked. When the sugar is used up, the muscles, in a healthy body, drink in sugar from your blood. After exercising, the muscles continue to drink in glucose from your blood to replenish the glucose that was there before exercise.

When you have insulin resistance, glucose from your blood has difficulty getting inside your muscles; the muscles act like a brick wall. As you begin to use and tone your muscles, they become more receptive to the glucose in your blood, allowing the glucose in. Studies show that the muscles specifically worked out in a given exercise take up glucose far more easily than another muscle in the same body, which has not been worked out. People with high blood sugar prior to muscle toning will find that their blood sugar levels are lower after the muscle has been worked.

On the downside, if you have normal blood sugar levels prior to working a muscle, you may find that your blood sugar goes too low after you exercise unless you eat something; this food should be carbohydrates. In fact, your muscles prefer to use carbohydrates rather than fat as fuel. When your muscles use up all the sugar in your blood, your liver will convert glycogen (excess glucose it stores up for these kinds of emergencies) back into glucose and release it into your bloodstream for your muscles to use.

To avoid this scenario, eat before and after exercising if your blood sugar level is normal. How much you eat prior to exercising largely depends on what you're doing and how long you're going to be doing it. The general rule is to follow your meal plan, eating smaller, more frequent meals throughout the day to keep your blood sugar levels consistent.

If your blood sugar is low, don't exercise at all, as doing so may be life-threatening. Do not resume exercise until you get your blood sugar levels under control.

exercises that can be hazardous

Exercises that can be hazardous, such as wrestling or weightlifting, are usually short but very intense. As a result, unless you fuel up ahead of time, these activities will force your body to use glycogen, which, as mentioned above, is the stored glucose your liver keeps handy. When you have diabetes, it's not a great idea to force your liver to give up that glycogen. This can actually increase your blood pressure and put you at risk for other health problems, including hypoglycemia. To avoid this, prior to doing these exercises, you'll need to eat some carbohydrates, which will provide enough fuel to the muscles.

eight

for your mental health

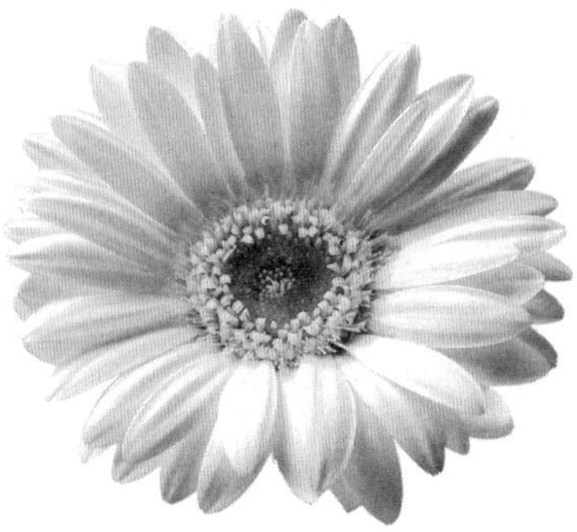

This chapter discusses the symptoms of depression, describes situations that can trigger depression, and offers reasons that some of us are more prone to depression than others.

In the majority of cases, women in their 50s suffering from depression have *unipolar depression*, a mood disorder characterized by one low mood. This is distinct from *bipolar depression*, a mood disorder in which there are two moods: one high mood and one low mood, normally diagnosed earlier in life, in the sufferer's late 20s or early 30s.

Most cases of unipolar depression are caused by life events or circumstances. For this reason, the term "situational depression" is used by mental health care experts to describe most cases of mild, moderate, or even severe unipolar depression in women. Examples of a "life event" that can trigger depression include: illness; loss of a loved one (the relationship may have ended, or a loved one may have died); reproductive life change (childbirth, hysterectomy, or menopause); job loss or change; or moving.

Situational depression can also be triggered by the *absence* of change in your life, meaning that you are living in a state of "continuous struggle," unhappiness or stress in which no light appears at the end of the tunnel. Examples include: chronic illness; abusive relationships; poverty or economic worries; job stress; or body image problems, such as feeling fat or unattractive.

A third catalyst for situational depression is an absence of resolution regarding past traumas and abuses. Examples include: sexual abuse; incest; violence; rape; or emotional abuse.

are you depressed or just sad?

Everyone experiences sadness, bad days, and bad moods. Feeling sad is not the same thing as feeling depressed. The first order of business, then, is to define what normal sadness is, and how it is distinct from depression. If you're unclear whether you're "just sad" or depressed, remember this: if you think you may be depressed, this is a good enough reason to seek help, even if you are not exhibiting the symptoms of depression discussed in this chapter.

sadness versus depression

Okay, remember this like a mantra: Sadness *lifts*, depression *persists*. That's how you can tell if you're just feeling sad, or are actually depressed. Feelings of sadness and grief (see below) are definitely common and normal in an infinite variety of circumstances. And, again, the symptoms of sadness often mirror those of depression: you're crying; you can't sleep; you can't eat. Eventually, however, as time passes, and you find yourself going back to your routine, the sadness *lifts*. You may still be sad or grieving, but you can also enjoy your life and put your unhappy thoughts on the back burner. That's not to say that the problem disappears, but you will be able to cope, with the right support. You may need to talk about your problem or life event to friends or family, but every day gets easier. You can get out of bed and have appreciation for something in life, whether it's a nice day, a good movie, or a delicious dessert.

When you're depressed, nothing lifts, and life gets more difficult, grayer, bleaker, until you begin to feel numb, and what you once found pleasurable no longer interests you. Your ability to function decreases with each passing day when you're depressed; your ability to function increases with each passing day when you're just sad about something. But the trigger—the event that has caused you to be sad or depressed—is always real, understandable, and legitimate. Never forget that.

What is tricky about the sadness versus depression question is that what triggered your sadness can also trigger a depression. Again, when the symptoms persist rather than lift, you are not getting better, and may need some help. (For a list of professionals who can help, see pages 189–191.)

grieving versus depression

One of the most common causes of sadness and suffering is grief. If you're grieving the loss of a loved one, and profound feelings of sadness, inability to eat, sleep, or concentrate persist beyond three months, your grief may have developed into a full-blown depression.

Because statistically women outlive their spouses more often than men do, women tend to suffer from grief more often. And about 10 per cent of all people who suffer the loss of a loved one require treatment for depression. There are certain people more likely to become depressed after a loss: people with a history of depression, people who have lost a relationship of many years, and people who have lost a relationship that was unresolved, creating profound feelings of guilt and regret. When a depression is triggered by grief, there are likely feelings of self-worth that are connected to your loss, which the depression may be bringing to the surface.

It's important to remember that you can also grieve for the loss of someone still very much alive. When you experience the end of a relationship or friendship with someone, feelings of grief over the loss of that relationship are similar to feelings of grief experienced when someone dies.

The human-animal bond is a powerful one, and the death of a pet can cause profound feelings of grief. Because of embarrassment over the feelings we have for our pets, however, many of us are afraid to admit or express grief over the loss. For many women, pets are real companions who offer unconditional acceptance and love. Pets often serve as vessels for many emotions that are never released into relationships with members of our own species.

And people are often guilt-ridden over having their pets euthanized, which adds another dimension to the grieving.

Grief has progressed to depression when: your grief persists longer than three months; you feel like dying or are suicidal; you are experiencing hallucinations or delusions (for example, you may see your deceased loved one or believe that person is still alive); you feel depressed every day, and have experienced the symptoms of depression discussed below for more than a month; you aren't caring for yourself (for example, you're not eating, bathing, and so on).

depression

Depression is clinically known as a mood disorder. It's impossible to define what a "normal mood" is since we all have such complex personalities, and exhibit different moods throughout a given week, or even a given day. However, it's not impossible for you to define what a "normal" mood is for *you*. You know how you feel when you're functional: you're eating, sleeping, interacting with friends and family, being productive, active, and generally interested in the daily goings-on of life. When you're depressed, you feel you've lost the ability to function for a prolonged period of time, or if you're functioning at a reasonable level to the outside world, you've lost interest in participating in life.

One bad day, or even a bad week (which will usually be made up of some relief time when you can laugh at something or take pleasure in something), from time to time, is not a sign that you're depressed. Feeling you've lost the ability to function as you *normally* do, all day, every day, for a period of at least two weeks, may be a sign that you're depressed.

The symptoms of depression vary from person to person, but can include some or all of the following:

- Feelings of sadness and "empty mood"
- Difficulty sleeping (usually waking up frequently in the middle of the night)
- Loss of energy and feelings of fatigue and lethargy
- Change in appetite (usually a loss of appetite)
- Difficulty thinking, concentrating, or making decisions
- Loss of interest in formerly pleasurable activities (anhedonia), including sex

- Anxiety or panic attacks
- Obsessing over negative experiences or thoughts
- Feeling guilty, worthless, hopeless, or helpless
- Feeling restless and irritable
- Thinking about death or suicide

when you can't sleep

The typical sleep pattern of a depressed person is to go to bed at the normal time, only to wake up around two in the morning and find that getting back to sleep is impossible. Endless hours are spent watching television to pass the time, or tossing and turning in bed, usually obsessing over negative experiences or thoughts. Lack of sleep affects the ability to function, and leads to increased irritability, lack of energy, and fatigue.

Insomnia, by itself, is not a sign of depression, but when you consider depression to be a package of symptoms, the inability to fall or stay asleep can aggravate all your other symptoms. In some cases, people who are depressed oversleep, requiring 10–12 hours of sleep every night.

when you can't think clearly

Another debilitating feature of depression is the inability to concentrate or think clearly. You feel scattered, disorganized, and unable to prioritize. This usually hits hardest in the workplace or school, and can severely impair job performance. You may miss deadlines and important meetings, or find you can't focus when you *do* go to meetings. When you can't think clearly, you can be overwhelmed with feelings of helplessness or hopelessness. "I can't even perform a simple task such as X anymore" may dominate your thoughts, while you become more disillusioned with your dwindling productivity.

anhedonia: when nothing gives you pleasure

One of the most conspicuous signs of depression is a loss of interest in activities that used to excite you or give you pleasure. This is known as *anhedonia*, derived from the word "hedonism," meaning the "philosophy of pleasure." Anhedonia simply means "no pleasure."

Different people have different ways of expressing anhedonia. You might tell your friends, for example, that you don't "have any desire" to do X or Y; you can't "get motivated"; or X or Y just doesn't "hold your interest or attention." You may also notice that the sense of satisfaction from a job well done is gone, which is particularly debilitating in the workplace or in a school. Artists may find the passion has gone out of their work.

Many of the other symptoms of depression hinge on this loss of pleasure. One of the reasons weight loss is so common in depression—typically, people may notice as much as a 10 pound drop in weight—is that food no longer gives them pleasure, or cooking no longer gives them pleasure. The sense of satisfaction we get from having a tidy home or clean kitchen may also disappear. Therefore, tackling cleaning up our kitchens in order to prepare food may be too taxing, contributing to a lack of interest in food.

Just as gaining weight is not an unusual symptom of depression, losing weight can occur as a result of depression, too. This is often due to poor nutrition as well: because we're not eating properly, we will fill up on snack foods or high-calorie, low-nutrient foods because we're not motivated to prepare or eat well-balanced meals. Weight gain may come from a loss of interest in physical activities: exercising, sports, or a dozen other things that keep us active when we're feeling "ourselves."

A loss of interest in sex aggravates matters if we are in a sexual relationship with someone. Again, the decreased desire for sex stems from general anhedonia.

causes of depression

Since most episodes of depression are triggered by life events or circumstances, the causes of depression are different for everyone. In a very general way, difficult circumstances cause depression. Understanding what's "difficult," however, is akin to understanding pain thresholds. What one woman finds difficult, another may not.

What we also know is that depression is on the rise—or at least, the *diagnosis* of depression is on the rise. As in other illnesses or diseases, when there is awareness and active screening for a condition (in this case, active screening is done through the diagnostic criteria listed in the DSM IV, which stands for *Diagnostic and Statistical Manual of Mental Disorders, 4th Edition*, an often-criticized "recipe book" on psychiatric symptoms, compiled by the American Psychiatric Association), there is a rise in its incidence. In other words, when you're looking for something, you'll find it. Of course, *not* looking for something doesn't mean it isn't there. The question remains: Is it better to seek out depression and treat it, ending unnecessary suffering? Many health care practitioners would answer in the affirmative.

Although there is some agreement that depression is a biological state, in that, yes, brain chemistry is altered in depressed people, it is unusual for this to occur in the absence of an environmental trigger, that is, a life event or chronic situation. This can be an actual emotional trauma, such as a divorce or death; unresolved traumas from the past that got buried; repressed anger (a significant contributing factor for women); workplace stress; physical illness, and a million other things. As mentioned earlier, when a life event triggers depression, mental health care experts refer to this as situational depression (also known as reactive or precipitated depression).

some depressing circumstances

It's useful to look at the life events that are common triggers of situational depression in women. Many of the symptoms of depression are understandable and logical, given some of the situations described below; in other words, you'd be crazy *not* to be depressed. The following is designed to give you a comprehensive view of women's experiences. (I've left birthdays off the list, but they are frequent triggers of depression because they represent aging, feelings of loss of beauty, vitality, and power. Difficult birthdays are typically ones that end in "5" or "0"—particularly the one that starts with 5 and ends in 0!)

Violence. One of the most identifiable "difficult circumstances" is violence. While statistics vary, as a result of the underreporting of violence, three out of four women will be victims of at least one violent crime during their lifetimes. In 1998, the number of women abused by their husbands was greater than the number of women who got married. Experts on domestic violence report that these assaults range from physical and sexual to verbal, can have many perpetrators, but usually men with whom there are relationships of trust are the assaulters: fathers, uncles, cousins, brothers, boyfriends, husbands, and so on.

Poverty. Single women and women of colour are far more likely to live in poverty than Caucasian men. After a divorce, a man's income increases by roughly 20 per cent , yet a women's income decreases by at least 50 per cent. Difficulty with paying bills and making ends meet leads to feelings of anxiousness, sleeplessness, stress, guilt, irritability, and persistent physical symptoms. And poverty is tiring: many women need to work at two or three jobs in order to survive, and cannot afford some of the conveniences that make life easier. This can result in fatigue, loss of energy, and loss of appetite, among other things.

Women in debt is a new spin on poverty; the poverty is often hidden by women who are living in seemingly comfortable surroundings, even though they have maxxed out their credit cards to pay the rent in between jobs or contracts; are being harassed by creditors; and are one day away from having their cars repossessed.

It's important to note that many women in poverty or debt are also the "hidden homeless." Untold numbers of women camp out on the couches of friends and relatives, while looking for employment or a place to live.

Workplace stress and/or harassment. Even though it's the 21st century, women still must cope with sexual harassment, ageism, and sexism in the workplace, which often leads to loss of employment. And women who are forced to work two jobs to make ends meet can be exposed to twice the abuse on the job in the form of harassment or stress, as well as the plain old stress caused by the long hours and commuting all people in the workplace endure.

Beauty standards. Impossible standards of beauty are another factor that makes life difficult for women. Aside from body image anxiety (see chapter 3), the physical symptoms caused by any resulting eating disorder can cause restlessness, irritability, difficulty concentrating or making decisions, loss of interest in formerly pleasurable activities, feelings of self-doubt, and self-hatred.

Hormonal factors. Hormonal changes related to perimenopause could certainly be looked upon as organic causes of depression, in that hormones can alter behaviour and moods, but many women argue that there are social stigmas attached to menopause, which cannot be ignored. Heavy, crampy periods or an unexpected period (due to the unpredictability of menopausal changes) in the middle of a busy workday are not insignificant stresses. Menopause is a social symbol of aging in Western culture, which in itself, has a number of powerful feelings associated with it (see chapter 1).

Illness. A related factor in many cases of depression is chronic illness. Women living with arthritis, osteoporosis, cancer, and other chronic diseases can experience many of the symptoms associated with depression, such as loss of appetite, sleeplessness, and loss of interest in formerly pleasurable activities. To aggravate matters, medications can cause depression as well.

Divorce. Whether you were living common-law or were married, the dissolution of a long-term relationship with an intimate partner leads to feelings of grief, sadness, loneliness, isolation, and often financial hardship: all fodder for depression.

when depression is a symptom of a physical ailment

Sometimes the signs of depression are actually symptoms of an underlying chronic illness or condition, such as chronic fatigue syndrome, thyroid disorders, environmental or stress-related illnesses, or SAD—seasonal affective disorder, a kind of depression that is caused by a lack of sunlight. In these cases, depression is not triggered by a life event or life situations, but by something purely organic, or physical.

the genetic link

With so many likely triggers to depression, it's logical to ask: "Why isn't *everyone* depressed, then? *Why me?*"

Some researchers believe that people have a genetic predisposition to depression. For example, let's say you had a genetic predisposition to lung cancer. If you never smoked, chances are, you wouldn't develop lung cancer. But if you smoked, you could potentially trip the lung cancer switch. Meanwhile, if you didn't have a genetic predisposition to lung cancer, you could smoke a pack of cigarettes each day until you were 90 and still never develop lung cancer. It works the same way with depression. The "cigarettes" in this case are difficult life circumstances, unforeseen stresses and tragedies, and other random acts of misfortune. Some of these circumstances we can control; other times, these circumstances are beyond our control, requiring us to tap into inner strengths, belief systems, and coping skills.

There are many who criticize genetic research into depression. While no specific gene has been found for depression, the hunt is definitely on, and it is a potentially dangerous hunt. Although it's clear to researchers that depression has many causes, and no one gene will likely be found to "cause" various kinds of depression, the worry is that once certain genes are even linked to depression, it may be easy to lose sight of the environmental triggers. In other words, instead of trying to enact legislation that may protect women from, say, domestic violence—a major trigger for depression—more emphasis will be placed on altering the battered woman's brain chemistry with drugs than on helping her to leave her abusive environment.

Furthermore, who will control the social harms associated with "depression genes"? What if we find that some minority or ethnic groups have more depression genes than other groups? This could potentially blacklist them from certain kinds of jobs, and so on. What if women are offered a prenatal test for depression genes and are given the opportunity to terminate pregnancies for fetuses that test positive for them? Would that be a good thing? At this stage, these are unanswerable questions. The simple fact remains, however, that life is difficult, and some people have less support and poorer coping skills than others to get through difficult circumstances. They need to learn how to mange desprssion.

managing depression

When you're suffering from the symptoms of depression, the first order of business is to stop the suffering, and get you back to your functioning self again. Long-term strategies to prevent a recurrence will vary, depending on the circumstances of your depression, and the type of depression you're suffering from.

short-term solutions

There is no one way to stop the suffering in depression. Different approaches work for different women. Some do well with talk therapy, others with drug therapy, and still others with a combination of the two.

talk therapy

Less invasive solutions to depression involve finding someone to talk to, which involve the following professionals:

- Psychiatrist. This is a doctor who specializes in the medical treatment of mental illness, and is able to prescribe drugs. Many psychiatrists also do psychotherapy, but this isn't always the case. The appropriate credentials should read: Jane Doe, M.D. (medical doctor), F.R.C.P. (Fellow, Royal College of Physicians). That means this doctor has gone through four years of medical school, and has completed a residency program in psychiatry, which, depending on the province, lasted approximately four years, and is registered in the Royal College of Physicians and Surgeons.
- Psychologist and Psychological Associate. This is someone who can be licensed to practice therapy with either a master's degrees or doctoral degree. Clinical psychologists have a Master of Science degree (M.Sc.) or Master of Arts (M.A.), and will usually work in a hospital or clinic

setting, but often can be found in private practice. Clinical psychologists can also hold a Ph.D. (Doctor of Philosophy) in psychology, an Ed.D. (Doctor of Education) or, if they're American, a Psy.D. (Doctor of Psychology), a common degree in the United States.

Psychologists should be registered in the College of Psychologists. In most provinces, someone calling him/herself a psychologist would have to be registered or licensed by a provincial body, which isn't necessarily meaningful unless the psychologist worked in a certain kind of setting. The problem with licences is that you could have someone who is well trained as a psychotherapist, with a Ph.D. in psychology, who isn't registered with the province; while someone with no training, who is an experimental psychologist, for example, having, say, spent most of his or her professional life working with white mice, could call himself/herself registered. Psychologists often perform testing, assessments, and plan treatments. They can also do psychotherapy, and may have hospital admitting privileges. In some states in the U.S., psychologists can also prescribe drugs. This is helpful to know in case you seek out help while spending time or living in the United States.

- Social Worker: This professional holds a BSW (Bachelor of Social Work), and/or an MSW (Master of Social Work), having completed a bachelor's degree in another discipline (which is not at all uncommon). Some social workers have a Ph.D. as well. The designation CSW stands for Certified Social Worker, which is given by the College of Social Work to say that this person is certified and meets the standards to be a member of the College. In order to obtain a CSW, exams and supervision are required. Social workers can provide counselling and psychotherapy, but it's important to ask your social worker what specific training he or she has had in the area of mental health.
- Psychiatric Nurse: This is most likely a registered nurse (R.N.) with a Bachelor of Science in nursing (B.Sc.) (which isn't absolutely required) who probably has, but doesn't necessarily require, a master's degree in nursing, too. The master's degree could be either an M.A. (Master of Arts) or an M.Sc. (Master of Science). This professional has done most of his or her training in a psychiatric setting, and may be trained to do psychotherapy.

- Counsellor: This professional has usually completed certification courses in counselling, and therefore has obtained a licence to practice psychotherapy; this person may have, but does not require, a university degree. Frequently, though, counsellors will have a master's degree in a related field, such as social work. Or, they may have a master's degree in a field that has nothing to do with mental health. The bad news is, there are no official credentials required by a counsellor, in that there is no legal regulation of the term. Nevertheless, while a television repair person can, in theory, legally set up a counselling practice, it's unlikely you'll encounter this.

  There are various provincial societies and associations to which counsellors may belong, but association, membership, or affiliation has little to do with this professional's skill as a therapist. For example, a counsellor's business card in Toronto may state that she is a member of the Ontario Society of Psychotherapy. That doesn't mean that she is a good psychotherapist, but it does mean that there are some standards of practice that she is upholding in order to be a member. It's always a good idea to ask your counsellor what training he or she has had in the field of mental health.
- Marriage and Family Counsellor: This term is somewhat different than the broader "counsellor." This professional has completed rigorous training through certification courses in family therapy and relationship dynamics, has obtained a licence to practise psychotherapy, and may or may not have a master's degree or Ph.D. in a related field. This professional should have the designations OAFMT or AAFMT.

Talk therapy may work best in combination with: herbal remedies (see What To Eat at the end of the chapter, and appendix C) and antidepressants. Antidepressants work on your brain chemistry. There are several types of prescription antidepressants, known as heterocyclics, monamine oxidase inhibitors (MOIs), and selective seritonin reuptake inhibitors (SSRIs). A subtype of SSRIs, called MSRIs, which stands for mixed seretonin reuptake inhibitors, is also popular, and includes seritonin-norepinephrine reuptake inhibitors (SNRIs). There are other kinds of antidepressants used as well, shown in Table 8.1.

TABLE 8.1: MEET YOUR ANTIDEPRESSANT

Monoamine oxidase inhibitors (MAOIs)

Common Side Effects: High/low blood pressure (this may cause dizziness); drowsiness, dry mouth; constipation. These drugs should not be used with over-the-counter cold and allergy medications, anti-diabetic drugs, narcotic painkillers, tricyclic antidepressants (unless the person is already on the tricyclic when starting this drug) or any SSRI.

Generic Name	Brand Name
phenelzine sulphate	Nardil®
tranylcypromine	Parnate®

Tricyclic antidepressants (TCAs)

Common Side Effects: These vary between sedation or agitation, depending on the brand. Other common side effects include: weight gain, dry mouth, blurry vision, low blood pressure, and sexual dysfunction (decreased interest in sex, problems with erection, and inability to achieve orgasm in both women and men). Tricyclics should not be taken with narcotic painkillers, MAOIs (unless you are already on the MAOI when you begin the trycyclic), and should only be combined with SSRIs with careful monitoring.

Generic Name	Brand Name
desipramine	Norpramin®
imipramine	Tofranil®
amitriptyline	Elavil®
nortriptyline	Aventyl®
doxepin	Sinequan®
trimipramine	Surmontil®
clomipramine	Anafranil®
maprotiline	Ludiomil®
protriptyline	Triptil
amoxapine	Asendin®
trazodene	Desyrel®

SSRIs (Selective seritonin reuptake inhibitors)

Common Side Effects: Sexual dysfunction such as the inability to achieve orgasm (Luvox excepted), nausea, and other gastrointestinal discomfort, diarrhea, sleeplessness or insomnia, short-term memory loss, tremors, restlessness, muscle spasms and twitches, involuntary movements of the face, limbs, and trunk.

Generic Name	Brand Name
fluoxetine	Prozac®
sertraline	Zoloft®
paroxetine	Paxil®
fluvoxamine	Luvox®

SNRIs (Serotonin-norepinephrine reuptake inhibitors)

Common Side Effects: SSRI-like side effects including agitation, nausea, headache, and gastrointestinal problems. Can cause high blood pressure, too.

Generic Name	Brand Name
venlafaxine	Effexor®
nefazodone	Serzone®

RIMAs (Reversible inhibitors of monoamine oxidase A)

Common Side Effects: headaches, sleep disturbances, dizziness, tremors, increased agitation or anxiety, gastrointestinal problems, heart palpitations, low blood pressure, dry mouth. Not to be combined with other tricyclic antidepressants.

Generic Name	Brand Name
moclobemide	Manerix

talking versus drugs

A common scenario for many women is to go through talk therapy for years without any real progress. This raises the issue of whether talk therapy alone is less effective than medications, or less effective than the combination of medications and talk therapy. (Of course, it can simply mean that the woman is with the wrong therapist!) The opposite scenario is medication without any talk therapy, which is not good either. The experts consulted for this book agreed that in cases of severe depression, a combination of medication and talk therapy was best. In cases where you're dealing with a particular crisis, or in mild to moderate depression, talk therapy alone has been shown to be very helpful. For example, in some studies, cognitive therapy (how the mind acquires, interprets, and makes judgments about information) is shown to be just as valuable a treatment for mild to moderate depression as antidepressants.

Most mental health professionals concur that if you've never experienced depression before, are not severely depressed, aren't suffering from any major physical symptoms, such as sleep disturbances or appetite problems, then talk therapy without medication is certainly worthwhile. If you don't seem to be improving after having been in therapy for four to six months, it's time to ask yourself whether you're with the right therapist, and whether you may benefit from another approach.

long-term solutions

Preventing a recurrence of a depressive episode involves prolonged therapy: long-term counselling or psychotherapy instead of short-term; long-term talk therapy in combination with medications or herbs; lifestyle changes (ranging from stress reduction techniques to dramatic changes involving residence, jobs, and relationships). Since long-term solutions often involve making dramatic changes in lifestyle, which can take a long time to come to terms with or to implement, counselling is often a key component in managing depression.

The "sharing" approach has been shown to be highly beneficial, particularly in cases where women share difficult circumstances or have difficulties in common. Professionals who provide counselling for women report that the support and confidence gained from other women, including woman-centred counselling, is very helpful.

This isn't true only for depression. Several studies have shown the value of support groups and support systems in treating many physical diseases, such as cancer. Since depression has so many causes, support groups for "depressed women" are not as useful as support groups for, say, women who are living with violence, or women who are battling obesity. In other words, finding or establishing a group of women who share your circumstances is the key to finding good support. Otherwise, you may wind up in a group where your circumstances are not understood at all. For example, if you were going through a divorce, someone coping with cancer may find your circumstances not "reason enough" for you to feel depressed. Or, someone with AIDS may find someone with a treatable cancer unreasonable in her feelings of depression. And so on.

Community and cultural norms are also a huge factor in finding the right support group. For example, Caucasian women may cope differently with depression than African-American or Hispanic women. East Indian women may cope differently than Asian women, while African-American women may cope differently than Caribbean or Somali women.

Where do you look for support? If you're struggling with making ends meet, for example, you won't likely find an ad in the paper inviting "All Poor Women" to a support group. But if you live in an economically disadvantaged community, responding to community-based programs, ranging from crafts groups to yoga, is the way to support. In fact, community outreach workers use arts and crafts, fitness, computer classes, and so on, as a tool to attract women within the community who could benefit from support. In community-based programs there is often a great deal of talking and sharing during, prior to, and after the activity. These are places where you make friends, find someone you can talk to, and most importantly, find that you're not alone in your situation.

what to eat

We now know there are a variety of daily nutrients that help to regulate our moods. Tryptophan, for example, which is found in milk and other dairy products, helps our bodies to build neurotransmitters, such as serotonin. Tryptophan is sometimes used separately as an "augmenter," to boost the effect of antidepressant medication.

The B vitamins are also important for mental health. Vitamin B_{12} is crucial for good general health, while other B-complex vitamins (thiamine, riboflavin, niacin, pyridoxine, pantothenic acid, and biotin) are essential for brain function, enabling you to be cognizant and alert. Food sources of B vitamins are: lean meats, whole grains, liver, seeds, nuts, wheat germ, and dairy products.

Folate, or folic acid, is particularly important for a healthy mood. It is found in liver, eggs, leafy greens, yeast, legumes, whole grains, nuts, fruits (bananas, orange juice, grapefruit juice), vegetables (broccoli, spinach, asparagus, Brussels sprouts). When you don't have enough "brain foods," you can become more prone to depression.

Calcium and magnesium are also linked to mood. Both of these nutrients aid your brain to transmit nerve impulses properly. Calcium is found in dairy products, leafy greens, eggs, and fish (particularly salmon and sardines); soy, nuts, whole grains, milk, meat, and fish contain magnesium. (For more about vitamins and minerals, see appendix C.)

carbohydrates and moods

One of the most important factors in diet and moods is blood sugar level. Many women, for example, find they suffer from repeated episodes of low blood sugar, known as hypoglycemia. This is usually caused by consuming too many carbohydrates, which produces an initial rush of energy, followed by a tremendous crash, which is sometimes known as postprandial depression (or postmeal depression). In fact, during episodes of depression, it's not unusual to crave simple carbohydrates, such as sugars and sweets. The simpler the carbohydrate, the faster it breaks down into glucose, and the faster the drop in blood sugar, which leads, in turn, to a drop in mood. People with seasonal affective disorder (SAD) are known to especially crave sugars, such as chocolate and candy. The cravings for sweets are so powerful in SAD (80 per cent of those with SAD experience these cravings), that many doctors consider it a symptom of SAD.

If you think you suffer from low blood sugar, schedule an appointment with a nutritionist through your doctor and plan a diet that is based on a variety of foods, rather than on one that is mostly carbohydrates. By increasing your intake of protein and fibre, you can help to delay the breakdown of your food into glucose, which will keep your blood sugar levels more stable throughout the day.

mood herbs

Mood and nerve herbs are selling faster than any other herb on the market. The following herbs can help to alleviate mild to moderate depression:

st. john's wort

St. John's wort (*Hypericum perforatum*) has been used as a nerve tonic in folk medicine for centuries. The herb has been shown to successfully treat mild to moderate depression and anxiety. It's been used in Germany for years as a first-line treatment for depression, and is endorsed by the American Psychiatric Association. Indeed, in Germany and other parts of Europe, it outsells Prozac® prescriptions. Since St. John's wort was introduced into North America in the early 1990s, millions have been successfully treated for depression with it. According to *Nutrition Business Journal*, in the United States, sales of St. John's wort and other botanical products reached an estimated $4.3 billion dollars in 1998.

St. John's wort has minimal side effects, can be mixed with alcohol, is nonaddictive, and the dosage does not need to be increased with antidepressants. Moreover, you can go on and off St. John's wort as you wish, without any problem; it helps you sleep and dream; it doesn't have any sedative effect, and in fact, enhances your alertness. Finally, it doesn't put you at risk for agitation, also known as hypomania.

The downside of St. John's wort is that there is a longer lag time before you feel its effects compared to prescription antidepressants, which means that the herb may not work well in severe depression. It can also make you oversensitive to sunlight, and may have some gastrointestinal side effects, such as nausea, loss of appetite, or abdominal pains. Experts advise that taking the herb with meals will alleviate the latter problem. Some people are also allergic to St. John's wort, and can develop skin rashes.

kava root

From the black pepper family, another popular herb is kava (*Piper methysticum*), which has been a popular herbal drink in the South Pacific for centuries. Kava grows on the islands of Polynesia, and is known to calm nerves, ease stress, fatigue, and anxiety, which results in an antidepressant effect.

Kava can also help alleviate migraine headaches and menstrual cramps. Placebo-controlled studies conducted by the National Institute of Mental Health showed that kava significantly relieved anxiety and stress, without the problem of dependency or addiction to the herb.

Kava should not be combined with alcohol because it can make the effects of alcohol more potent. You should also check with your doctor before you combine kava with any prescription medications.

SAM-e

Sam-e (pronounced "Sammy") stands for S-adenosylmethionine, a compound made by your body's cells shown to help alleviate depression in mild to moderate cases. Since it was introduced in the United States in March 1999, more people have purchased SAM-e than St. John's wort. One reason could be that SAM-e helps to relieve joint pain and improve liver function, which makes it popular for people who suffer from arthritis as well as depression.

Studies done in Italy during the 1970s documented SAM-e's effectiveness as an antidepressent; recent U.S. studies confirm these results. Right now, psychiatrists are endorsing the use of SAM-e in cases of mild to moderate depression. Similar to the effects of antidepressants, however, some SAM-e users experience mild mania. Some people have also reported hot, itchy ears as a side effect.

other natural compounds

A variety of other compounds have been linked to combatting depression, or some of its features, such as sleeplessness or stress. These include:

- Gamma-aminobutyric acid (GABA). This is an amino acid that is supposedly an anti-anxiety agent, which may also help you to fall asleep if you suffer from sleeplessness.
- Inositol. This is a naturally occurring antidepressant that is present in many foods, such as vegetables, whole grains, milk, and meat, and is available over the counter.
- Dehydroepiandrosterone (DHEA). This is a hormone produced by the adrenal glands; production declines as we age. In certain studies, it has been shown to improve moods and memory, it is not yet available in Canada.
- Melatonin. This is a hormone that improves sleep and helps reset the body's natural clock. It is not yet available in Canada.
- Phosphatidylserine (PS). This is a phospholipid, a substance that feeds brain cell membranes. Studies show that it has natural antidepressant qualities.
- Tetrahydrobiopterin (BH4). This substance activates enzymes that control serotonin, noradrenaline, and dopamine levels, which are all important for stable moods. Some studies show that BH4 is an effective natural treatment for depression.

- Phenylethylamine (PEA). This is a nitrogen-containing compound found in small quantities in the brain. Studies show that it works as a natural antidepressant.
- Rubidium. This is a natural chemical in our bodies, belonging to the same family as lithium, potassium, and sodium. Studies show that it can work as an antidepressant.
- Ginkgo. This is a plant used to treat a variety of ailments, and is a common herb in Chinese medicine. It can improve memory, and some studies show that it can boost the effectiveness of antidepressant medications
- Valerian Root. This is similar to kava root in that it works as an anti-anxiety agent. It is also useful in combatting insomnia.

how to move

Getting outdoors and exposing yourself to some real sunlight is the first step in managing depression or low moods. Fifteen minutes of sunlight on your uncovered eyelids (take out contact lenses) daily is the general recommendation.

Aerobic exercise produces endorphins, "feel good" hormones, which have been shown to decrease the incidence of depression. If you can't find the time or inclination to exercise, try to incorporate some activity into your day. Inactivity and sedentary living breeds depression and sadness. When you get up and do something, or see people, you feel more alive and part of this world.

Exercise also combats weight gain, which often occurs with depression, as you may turn to food for comfort. The more weight you gain, the more depressed you often feel, which fuels more comfort eating, and a worsening of depression. By following the How To Move tips in chapters 2 and 3, you can do wonders to combat depression and boost your mental health and well-being.

postures and stretches to improve tranquility

1. While sitting or standing, raise your arms above your head. Keep your shoulders relaxed and breathe deeply for 5 seconds. Release and repeat 5 times.

2. Gently raise your shoulders in an exaggerated shrug. Breathe deeply and hold for 10 seconds. Relax, and repeat 3 times.
3. Lotus. Sit cross-legged on the floor with spine straight and neck aligned (see figure i). Focus on your breath, letting it gently fill the diaphragm and the back of the rib cage. On the inhalation, say "So," and on the exhalation, say "Hum." Voicing the breath in this manner will keep you focused and relaxed. Continue with "So-Hum" until you feel at ease.

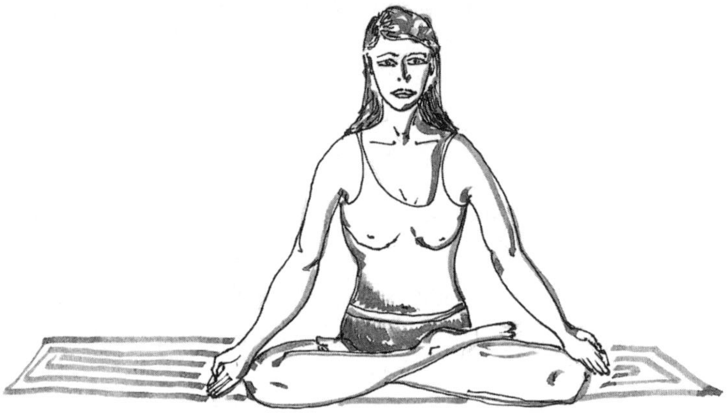

figure i

4. Child's Pose. Sit on your heels. Bring your forehead to the floor in front of you. Breathe into the back of the rib cage, feeling the stretch in your spine. Hold as long as it's comfortable.
5. Tree. Stand tall and focus on a point across the room. Place the heel of one foot on the opposite inner thigh. Float your arms upward until your palms are touching (see figure ii). Breathe deeply, and hold for 5 seconds. Release and repeat on the other side.

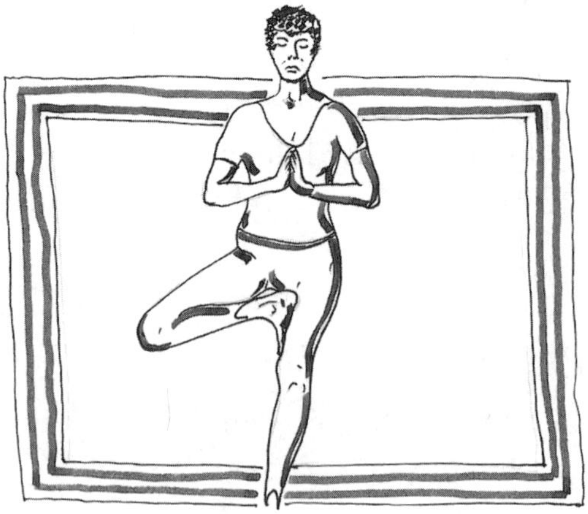

figure ii

6. Savasana or Corpse Pose. Lie on your back with palms facing upward, feet turned gently outward. Focus on the movement of breath throughout your body.
7. Bow. Lie on your belly, with arms at your sides. Bend your legs at the knees and bring your heels in toward your buttocks. Reach back and take hold of your right, then your left, ankle. Flex your feet if you're having a hard time maintaining this position. Inhale, raising the upper body as far off the floor as possible. Lift your head, completing the arch. Your knees should remain as close together as possible (tying them together might help here). Breathe deeply, and hold for 10–15 seconds.
8. Cobra. Lie on your belly with your palms down and adjacent to your shoulders (see figure iiia). Slowly raise your upper body, lifting all but the lower abdomen toward the ceiling (see figure iiib). Breathe deeply. Release.

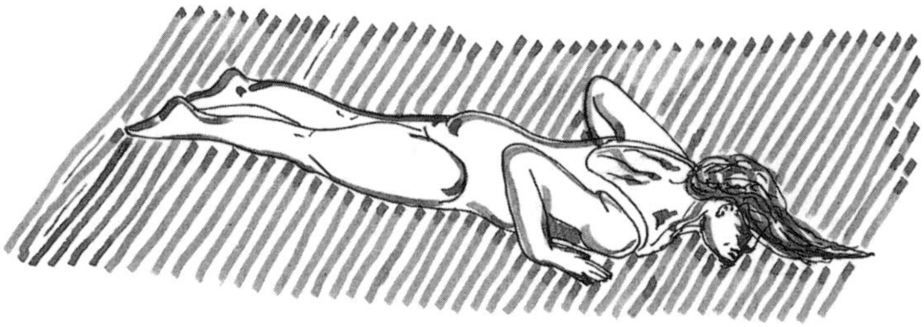

figure iiia

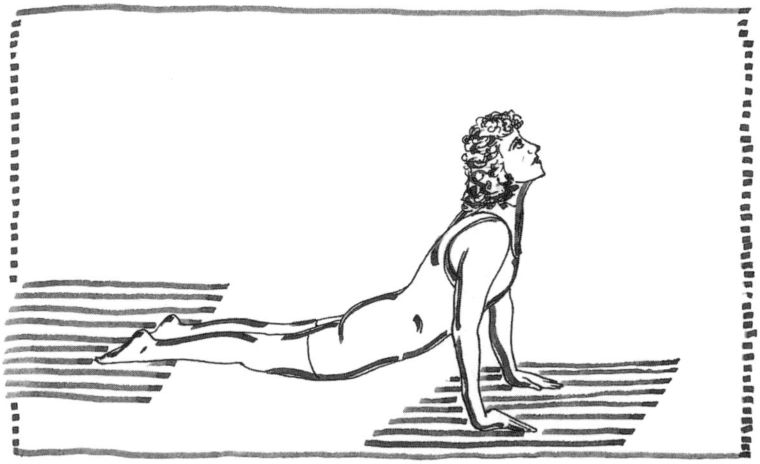

figure iiib

aromatherapy

Essential oils, made from plants, mostly herbs and flowers, can do wonders to relieve stress naturally; many essential oils are known for their calming and antidepressant effects.

The easiest way to use essential oils is in a warm bath. Add a few drops of the oil into your bath water. Sit and relax in it for about 10 minutes. Essential oils can also be inhaled (put a few drops in a bowl of hot water, lean over with a towel over your head, and breathe); diffused (using a lamp ring, or a ceramic diffuser—that thing that looks like a fondue pot); or sprayed into the air as a mist.

The following essential oils are known to have calming, sedative, or antidepressant effects: ylang ylang; neroli; jasmine; cedarwood; lavender (a few drops on your pillow will also help you sleep); chamomile; marjoram; geranium; patchouli; rose; sage; clary sage; and sandalwood.

APPENDIX A herbs for perimenopause

Black Cohosh (*Cimicifuga racemosa*), Schwarze Sclangenwurzel
(Chinese herbalists use Sheng Ma: *C. foetida, C. dahurica*)
Medicinal benefits:

- Reduces intensity and frequency of hot flashes
- Eases the general discomforts of menopause
- Tones and strengthens pelvic floor muscles, preventing and correcting uterine and bladder prolapses
- Improves digestion
- Relieves menstrual pain and irregularity
- Relieves headaches
- Relieves angina pain and thins the blood
- Calms the nerves
- Alleviates water retention and breast tenderness
- Aids with incontinence

Vitex or **Chaste Tree (*Vitex agnus-castii*)**
(Chinese herbalists use Man Jing Zi)

- Helps improve endometriosis and uterine fibroids
- Reduces severity of hot flashes
- Relieves chronic menstrual cramps
- Relieves heavy bleeding and spotting, and irregular cycles
- Calms the nerves
- Clears up skin problems
- Relieves hormone-related constipation and digestive problems
- Lessens breast tenderness
- Relieves water retention
- Relieves PMS symptoms
- Protects against reproductive cancers
- Protects against osteoporosis
- Treats vaginal infections

Liferoot (*Senecio aureus*)/Groundsel (*Senecio vulgaris*)/Jacob's Groundsel (*Senecio jacobaea*)

- Relieves severe menstrual pain
- Alleviates hot flashes
- Tones uterus
- Regulates the menstrual cycle
- Calms the nerves
- Relieve PMS symptoms and breast tenderness
- Reduces urinary tract problems
- Increases libido

Garden sage (*Salvia officinalis*), Salbei, Sauge officinale
Do not use: sagebrush/desert sage (*Artemisia tridentata*)

- Relieves night sweats, cold sweats, and hot-flash sweats
- Calms the nerves
- Relieves dizziness, trembling, and mood swings associated with profuse sweating
- Relieves headaches
- Strengthens the liver and aids digestion
- Relieves menstrual cramps and heavy bleeding
- Reduces bladder infections
- Prevents joint aches and increases circulation
- Improves mental clarity and memory

Motherwort (*Leonurus cardiaca*), Herzgespan, Yi Mu Cao

- Lessens the severity, frequency, and duration of hot flashes
- Relieves faintness associated with hot flashes
- Calms the nerves and helps lift depression
- Relieves insomnia and sleep disturbances

- Strengthens the heart, and reduces palpitations and tachycardia (abnormally rapid heart rate)
- Relieves menstrual cramps or uterine cramps
- Restores thickness and elasticity to vaginal walls
- Reduces water retention
- Relieves constipation and improves digestion

Ginseng

Oriental ginseng/Ren Shan (Panax ginseng)

American ginseng (*Panax quinquefolius*)

- Reduces the intensity and frequency of hot flashes
- Calms the nerves and lifts the mood
- Reduces stress
- Reduces heavy menstrual flow
- Improves overall energy levels and reduces fatigue
- Improves memory, concentration, mental acuity, and clarity
- Normalizes blood pressure and reduces cholesterol
- Stabilizes blood sugar swings
- Reduces headaches associated with menopause
- Improves digestion
- Enhances libido

Note: American ginseng is less potent than the ginseng grown in Korea and China.

Dang Gui (*Angelic sinensis*) or **Dong Quai**

- Relieves hot flashes
- Regulates the menstrual cycle (see note below)
- Relieves uterine cramps
- Helps reduce vaginal dryness and thinning
- Helps restore complexion
- Reduces headaches and water retention
- Reduces blood pressure and improves circulation (contains coumarins, like aspirin)
- Reduces insomnia
- Calms the nerves
- Relieves menopausal rheumatism
- Tones the liver

Note: Do not use Dang Gui if you have unpredictable episodes of heavy menstrual bleeding, fibroids, diarrhea, or edema, or if you regularly take aspirin or other blood-thinning drugs.

APPENDIX B herbs for postmenopause

Horsetail (*Equisetum arvense*)

- Reverses osteoporosis
- Stimulates fracture-mending and bone repair
- Stabilizes and reverses gum disease and loss of jawbone
- Relieves cystitis (bladder infection)
- Reduces bloat
- Improves circulation
- Increases energy, reduces fatigue
- Nourishes hair and fingernails

Oatstraw (*Avena sativa*)

(From the same oats you eat for breakfast)

- Helps build bones
- Maintains teeth
- Stabilizes blood sugar levels
- Relieves depression
- Reduces cholesterol
- Maintains restful sleep patterns
- Helps with bladder spasms, incontinence, uterine pain, and vaginal dryness

Seaweeds

- Helps prevent osteoporosis
- Lowers blood pressure and cholesterol
- Helps with varicose veins and hemorrhoids
- Nourishes the heart
- Relieves incontinence, vaginal dryness, and persistent hot flashes
- Increases immunity
- Increases stamina
- Minimize the effects of stress, chemicals, and radiation
- Improves digestion
- Restores libido
- Eases sore joints
- Nourishes skin and hair

Stinging Nettle (*Urtica dioica, Urtica urens*)

- Nourishes kidneys and adrenal glands
- Relieves bladder infections, bloat, and incontinence
- Rehydrates dry vaginal tissues
- Stabilizes blood sugar
- Reduces headaches
- Improves immunity
- Improves digestion
- Strengthens nervous system
- Nourishes cardiovascular system
- Nourishes skin and hair

Bioflavonoids

All foods and herbs rich in bioflavonoids will help to:

- Restore vaginal lubrication
- Improve pelvic tone
- Strengthen the bladder
- Reduce water retention
- Ease sore joints
- Improve hot flashes
- Improve liver activity
- Lower risk of stroke and heart attack
- Reduce muscle cramping
- Improve resistance to infection

Foods and herbs rich in bioflavonoids include:

- Citrus fruits
- Buckwheat greens, such as alfalfa sprouts
- Elder
- Hawthorn
- Knotweeds, Ho Shou Wu
- Roses
- Shepherd's purse
- Sea buckhorn
- Toadflax
- White dead nettle

APPENDIX C vitamins and minerals for 50-something

Bioflavonoids: Found in citrus pulp and rind. Herbal sources: buckwheat greens, blue green algae, elderberries, hawthorn fruits, rosehips, horsetail, shepherd's purse.

Boron: Found in organic fruits, vegetables, nuts. Herbal sources: all organic weeds including chickweed, purslane, nettles, dandelion, yellow dock.

Calcium: Found in milk and dairy products, leafy greens, broccoli, clams, oysters, almonds, walnuts, sunflower seeds, sesame seeds (e.g. tahini), legumes, tofu; softened bones of canned fish (sardines, mackerel, salmon), seaweed vegetables, whole grain, whey, shellfish. *Herbal sources*: valerian, kelp, nettle, horsetail, peppermint, sage, uva ursi, yellow dock, chickweed, red clover, oatstraw, parsley, blackcurrent leaf, raspberry leaf, plantain leaf/seed, borage, dandelion leaf, amaranth leaves, lamb's quarter. *Depleted by*: coffee, sugar, salt, alcohol, cortisone enemas, too much phosphorus.

Carotenes: Found in carrots, cabbage, winter squash, sweet potatoes, dark leafy greens, apricots, spirulina, seaweeds. *Herbal sources*: peppermint, yellow dock, uva ursi, parsley, alfalfa, raspberry leaves, nettle, dandelion greens, kelp, green onions, violet leaves, cayenne, paprika, lamb's quarter, sage, peppermint, chickweed, horsetail, black cohosh, rosehips.

Chromium: Found in barley grass, bee pollen, prunes, nuts, mushrooms, liver, beets, whole wheat. *Herbal sources*: oatstraw, nettle, red clover, catnip, dulse, wild yam, yarrow, horsetail, black cohosh, licorice, echinacea, valerian, sarsaparilla. *Depleted by*: white sugar.

Copper: Found in liver, shellfish, nuts, legumes, water, organically grown grains, leafy greens, seaweeds, bittersweet chocolate. *Herbal sources*: skullcap, sage, horsetail, chickweed.

Essential fatty acids (EFAs), including GLA, omega-6, and omega-3: Found in safflower oil, wheat germ oil. *Herbal sources*: all wild plants contain EFAs. *Commercial sources*: flaxseed oil, evening primrose, black current, and borage.

Folic acid (B factor): Found in liver, eggs, leafy greens, yeast, legumes, whole grains, nuts, fruits (bananas, orange juice, grapefruit juice), vegetables (broccoli, spinach, asparagus, Brussels sprouts). *Herbal sources*: nettle, alfalfa, parsley, sage, catnip, peppermint, plantain, comfrey leaves, chickweed.

Iron: (Heme iron is easily absorbed by the body; non-heme iron is not as easily absorbed, so should be taken with Vitamin C.) Heme iron is found in liver, meat, and poultry; non-heme iron is found in dried fruit, seeds, almonds, cashews, enriched and whole grains, legumes, green leafy vegetables. *Herbal sources*: chickweed, kelp, burdock, catnip, horsetail, Althea root, milk thistle seed, uva ursi, dandelion leaf/root, yellow dock, Dang Gui, black cohosh, echinacea, plantain leaves, sarsaparilla, nettle, peppermint, licorice, valerian, fenugreek. *Depleted by*: coffee, black tea, enemas, alcohol, aspirin, carbonated drinks, lack of protein, too much dairy.

Magnesium: Found in leafy greens, seaweeds, nuts, whole grains, yogurt, cheese, potatoes, corn, peas, squash. *Herbal sources*: oatstraw, licorice, kelp, nettle, dulse, burdock, chickweed, Althea root, horsetail, sage, raspberry leaf, red clover, valerian, yellow dock, dandelion, carrot tops, parsley, evening primrose. *Depleted by*: hot flashes, night sweats, crying jags, alcohol, chemical diuretics, enemas, antibiotics, excessive fat intake.

Manganese: Found in any leaf or seed from a plant grown in healthy soil; seaweeds. *Herbal sources*: raspberry leaf, uva ursi, chickweed, milkthistle, yellow dock, ginseng, wild yam, hops, catnip, echinacea, horsetail, kelp, nettle, dandelion.

Molybdenum: Found in organically raised dairy products, legumes, grains, leafy greens. *Herbal sources*: nettle, dandelion greens, sage, oatstraw, fenugreek, raspberry leaves, red clover, horsetail, chickweed, seaweeds.

Niacin (B factor): Found in grains, meats and nuts, and especially asparagus, spirulina, cabbage, bee pollen. *Herbal sources*: hops, raspberry leaf, red clover, slippery elm, echinacea, licorice, rosehips, nettle, alfalfa, parsley.

Nickel: Found in chocolate, nuts, dried beans, cereals. *Herbal sources*: alfalfa, red clover, oatstraw, fenugreek.

Phosphorus: Found in whole grains, seeds, nuts. *Herbal sources*: peppermint, yellow dock, milk thistle, fennel, hops, chickweed, nettle, dandelion, parsley, dulse, red clover. *Depleted by*: antacids.

Potassium: Found in bananas,celery, cabbage, peas, parsley, broccoli, peppers, carrots, potato skins, eggplant, whole grains, pears, citrus, seaweeds. *Herbal sources*: sage, catnip, hops, dulse, peppermint, skullcap, kelp, red clover, horsetail, nettle, borage, plantain. *Depleted by*: frequent hot flashes with sweating, night sweats, coffee, sugar, salt, alcohol, enemas, vomiting, diarrhea, chemical diuretics, dieting.

Pyridoxine (B_6): Found in baked potato with skin, broccoli, prunes, bananas, dried beans and lentils; all meats, poultry, fish.

Riboflavin (B_2): Found in beans, greens, onions, seaweeds, spirulina, dairy products, mushrooms. *Herbal sources*: peppermint, alfalfa, parsley, echinacea, yellow dock, hops; dandelion, ginseng, dulse, kelp, fenugreek.

Selenium: Found in dairy products, seaweeds, grains, garlic, liver, kidneys, fish, shellfish. *Herbal sources*: catnip, milk thistle, valerian, dulse, black cohosh, ginseng, uva ursi, hops, echinacea, kelp, raspberry leaf, rosebuds and rosehips, hawthorn berries, fenugreek, sarsaparilla, yellow dock.

Silicon: Found in unrefined grains, root vegetables, spinach, leeks. *Herbal sources*: horsetail, dulse, echinacea, cornsilk, burdock, oatstraw, licorice, chickweed, uva ursi, sarsaparilla.

Sulfur: Found in eggs, dairy products, cabbage family plants, onions, garlic, parsley, watercress. *Herbal sources*: nettle, sage, plantain, horsetail.

Thiamine (vitamin B_1): Found in asparagus, cauliflower, cabbage, kale, spirulina, seaweeds, citrus. *Herbal sources*: peppermint, burdock, sage, yellow dock, alfalfa, red clover, fenugreek, raspberry leaves, nettle, catnip, watercress, yarrow, briar rosebuds, rosehips

Vitamin A/Beta Carotene: Found in liver, fish oils, egg yolks, whole milk, butter; Beta Carotene—leafy greens, yellow and orange vegetables and fruits. *Depleted by*: coffee, alcohol, cortisone, mineral oil, fluorescent lights, liver "cleansing," excessive intake of iron, lack of protein.

Vitamin B_6: Found in meats, poultry, fish, nuts, liver, bananas, avocados, grapes, pears, egg yolk, whole grains, legumes.

Vitamin B_{12}: Found in meats, dairy products, eggs, liver, fish. *Both B_{12} and B_6 Depleted by*: coffee, alcohol, tobacco, sugar, raw oysters, birth control pills.

Vitamin C: Found in citrus fruits, broccoli, green pepper, strawberries, cabbage, tomato, cantaloupe, potatoes, leafy greens. *Herbal sources*: rosehips, yellow dock, raspberry leaf, red clover, hops, nettle, pine needles, dandelion greens, alfalfa, echinacea, skullcap, parsley, cayenne, paprika. *Depleted by*: antibiotics, aspirin and other pain relievers, coffee, stress, aging, smoking, baking soda, high fever.

Vitamin D: Found in fortified milk, butter, leafy green vegetables, egg yolk, fish oils, butter, liver, skin exposure to sunlight, shrimp. *Herbal sources*: not found in plants. *Depleted by*: mineral oil used on the skin, frequent baths, sunscreens with SPF 8 or higher.

Vitamin E: Found in nuts, seeds, whole grains, fish-liver oils, leafy greens, kale, cabbage, asparagus. *Herbal sources*: alfalfa, rosehips, nettle, Dang Gui, watercress, dandelions, seaweeds, wild seeds. *Depleted by*: mineral oil, sulphates.

Vitamin K: Found in leafy greens, corn and soybean oils, liver, cereals, dairy products, meats, fruits, egg yolk, blackstrap molasses. *Herbal sources*: nettle, alfalfa, kelp, green tea. *Depleted by*: X-rays, radiation, air pollution, enemas, frozen foods, antibiotics, rancid fats, aspirin.

Zinc: Found in oysters, seafood meat, liver, eggs, whole grains, wheat germ, pumpkin seeds, spirulina. *Herbal sources*: skullcap, sage, wild yam, chickweed, echinacea, nettle, dulse, milk thistle, sarsaparilla. *Depleted by*: alcohol and air pollution.

APPENDIX D where to go for more information

General Women's Health

The Canadian Women's Health Network
419 Graham Avenue, Suite 203
Winnipeg, MB R3C 0M3
Tel: (204) 942-5500
Fax: (204) 989-2355
Clearinghouse: 1-888-818-9172
e-mail: cwhn@cwhn.ca
Web site: www.cwhn.ca

The Centre for Research in Women's Health
790 Bay Street, 7th Floor
Toronto, ON M5G 1N8
Tel: (416) 351-3732
Fax: (416) 351-3746
e-mail: crwh.research@utoronto.ca
Web site: www.utoronto.ca/crwh and
www.womenshealthmatters.ca

Menopause

The Menopause Center
P.O. Box 1339
Squamish, WA 98392-1339
Tel: (360) 598-3688
e-mail: mtimes@telebyte.net

Note: This organization publishes the newsletter *MenoTimes*, published and edited by Brenda Beeley, a licensed acupuncturist, classical homeopath, and herbalist. She is a graduate of the Hahnemann College of Homeopathy and the San Francisco College of Acupuncture.

North American Menopause Society
(NAMS)
P.O. Box 94527
Cleveland, OH 44101
Tel: (216) 844-8748
e-mail:info@menopause.org
Web site: www.menopause.org

Breast Cancer

National

Alliance of Breast Cancer Survivors
P.O. Box 2035
20 Eglinton Avenue West
Toronto, ON M4R 1K8
Tel: (416) 487-9899
Fax: (416) 487-0584

Breast Cancer Action
P.O. Box 4332
Station E
Ottawa, ON K1S 5B3
Tel: (613) 736-5921

Breast Cancer Information Exchange
Project
Preventive Health Service Division
Health Canada
Jean Mance Building, Room 641
Tunney's Pasture
Ottawa, ON K1A 1B4
Tel: (613) 954-8668
Fax: (613) 941-2633

Breast Implant Line of Canada
56 Touraine Avenue
North York, ON M3H 1R2
Tel: (416) 636-6618

Canadian Breast Cancer Foundation
790 Bay Street, Suite 1000
Toronto, ON M5G 1N8
Tel: (416) 596-6773 or 1-800-387-9816

Canadian Breast Cancer Network
P.O. Box 39022
RPO Billings
Ottawa, ON K1H 1A1

Canadian Cancer Society
National Office
10 Alcorn Avenue, Suite 200
Toronto, ON M4V 3B1
Tel: (416) 961-7223
Fax: (416) 961-4189
Web site: www.cancer.ca

Canadian Palliative Care Association
R, 131C-43 Bruyere Street
Ottawa, ON K1N 5C8
Tel: 1-800-668-2785
Fax: (613) 241-3986
Web site: www.cpca.net

Ontario Cancer Treatment and Research Foundation
620 University Avenue, Suite 1500
Toronto, ON M5G 2L7
Tel: (416) 971-9800
Fax: (416) 971-6888
Web site: www.cancercare.on.ca

"Wellspring" (Support Group)
The Coach House
81 Wellesley Street East
Toronto, ON M4Y 1H6
Tel: (416) 961-1928
Fax: (416) 961-3721
Web site: www/wellspring.ca

Provincial Offices
Alberta / Northwest Territories
Alberta Cancer Board
9707–110 Street, 6th Floor
Edmonton, AB T5K 2L9
Tel: (403) 782-3491

Breast Cancer Info Link
1331-29 Street NW
Calgary, AB T2N 4N2
Tel: (403) 670-2113
Fax: (403) 270-8003

Canadian Cancer Society
2424–4th Street SW, Suite 2000
Calgary, AB T2S 2T4
Tel: (403) 228-4487

Cross Cancer Institute
11560 University Avenue
Edmonton, AB T6G 1Z2
Tel: (708) 432-8763
Web site: www.cancerboard.ab.ca

Prairies/NWT Breast Cancer Info Link
c/o Canadian Cancer Society
Alberta/NWT Division
2424-4th Street SW, Suite 200
Calgary, AB T2S 2T4
Tel: (403) 228-4487

Tom Baker Cancer Centre
1331–29th Street N.W.
Calgary, AB T2N 4N2
Tel: (403) 670-1711

British Columbia
B.C. Yukon Breast Cancer Information Project
c/o Canadian Cancer Society
B.C./Yukon Division
565 West 10th Avenue
Vancouver, BC V5Z 4J4
Tel: (604) 872-4400
Fax: (604) 879-4533
Web site: www.bc.cancer.ca

Cancer Control Agency of British Columbia
600 West 10th Avenue
Vancouver, BC V5Z 4E6
Tel: (604) 877-6000

Cancer Information Service
565 West 10th Avenue
Vancouver, BC V5Z 4J4
Tel: (604) 879-2323 or 1-888-939-3333
Fax: (604) 879-9267

Victoria Cancer Clinic
1900 Fort Street
Victoria, BC V8R 1J8

Manitoba
Canadian Cancer Society
193 Sherbrook Street
Winnipeg, MB R3C 2B7
Tel: (204) 774-7483
Fax: (204) 774-7500
e-mail: ccsman@gatewest.net

Manitoba Cancer Treatment and
Research Foundation
100 Olivia Street
Winnipeg, MB R3E 0V9
Tel: (204) 787-2271
e-mail: admin@mctrf.mb.ca

New Brunswick
Canadian Cancer Society
P.O. Box 2089
63 Union Street
Saint John, NB E2L 3T5
Tel: (506) 634-6272

Newfoundland and Labrador
Canadian Cancer Society
P.O. Box 8921
Crosby Building, 2nd Floor
St. John's, NF A1B 3R9
Tel: (709) 753-6520
Fax: (709) 753-9314
e-mail:ccfnf@thezone.net
Web site: www.nfandlab.cancer.ca

Newfoundland Cancer Clinic
Health Sciences Centre
Prince Philip Drive
St. John's, NF A1B 3V6
Tel: (709) 737-6439
e-mail: akwan@morgan.ucs.mun.ca

Newfoundland Cancer Treatment
and Research Foundation
25 Kenmount Road
St. John's, NF A1B 1W1

Nova Scotia
Canadian Cancer Society
5826 South Street, Suite 1
Halifax, NS B3H 1S6
Tel: (902) 423-6183
Fax: (902) 429-6563
e-mail: nstn3332@fox.nstn.ca

Cancer Center
QE2 Health Science Centre
5820 University Avenue
Halifax, NS B3H 1V7
Tel: (902) 473-6000

Ontario
Breast Cancer Information and
Education Services
366 Paul Street
St. Catharines, ON L2R 3N2
Tel: (905) 687-3333

Burlington Breast Cancer Support Service
777 Guelph Line
Burlington, ON L7R 3N2
Tel: (905) 634-2333
Web site: www.worldchat.com/web/bbcss
e-mail: bbcss@wchat.on.ca

Canadian Cancer Society
1639 Yonge Street
Toronto, ON M4T 2W6
Tel: (416) 488-5400
Web site: www.ontario.cancer.ca

Cancer Information Service
328 Mountain Park Avenue, 3rd Floor
Hamilton, ON L8V 4X2
Tel: 1-888-939-3333
Web site: www.cancer.ca

Ontario Breast Cancer Information
Exchange Pilot Project
c/o Toronto-Bayview Regional Cancer
Centre
2075 Bayview Avenue
Toronto, ON M4N 8M5
Tel: (416) 480-5899
Fax: (416) 480-6002

Thunder Bay Regional Cancer Centre
290 Munro Street
Thunder Bay, ON P7A 7T1
Tel: (807) 345-2030

Prince Edward Island

Atlantic Breast Cancer Information Project
1 Rochford Street, Suite 1
Charlottetown, PEI C1A 3T1
Tel: (902) 892-9531
Fax: (902) 628-8281

Canadian Cancer Society
1 Rochford Street, Suite 1
Charlottetown, PEI C1A 9L2
Tel: (902) 566-4007
Fax: (902) 429-6563

Quebec

Breast Cancer Action
5890 Monkland, Suite 203
Montreal, QC H4A 1G2
Tel: (514) 483-1846
Fax: (514) 482-1445

Canadian Cancer Society
5151, boul. l'Assomption
Montreal, QC H1T 4A9
Tel: (514) 255-5151
Web site: www.cancer.ca

Réseau d'échange l'information du Québec sur le cancer du sein/Quebec Breast Cancer Information Project
c/o Hotel-Dieu de Montréal
3840 rue St.-Urbain
Pavillion de Bullion, bureau 6-108
Montréal, QC H2W1T8
Tel: (514) 843-2930
Fax: (514) 843-2932
Web site: www.reiqcs.org

Tele Cancer/Infor Cancer
2075 Champlain Street
Montreal, PQ H2L 2T1
Tel: 1-800-363-0063

Saskatchewan

Allan Blair Memorial Clinic
4101 Dewdney Avenue
Regina, SK S4T 7T1
Tel: (306) 766-2213

Canadian Cancer Society
201–2445 13th Avenue
Regina, SK S4P 0W1
Tel: (306) 757-4260
Fax: (306) 569-2133

Breast Cancer Web sites

- American Cancer Society: www.cancer.org
- American Society of Clinical Oncology (ASCO): www.asco.org
- Canadian Cancer Society: www.cancer.ca
- Cancer Care: www/camcercareinc.org
- Educare: Cancer Help Breast Cancer: www.cancerhelp.com/ed
- Frontier Breast Cancer Fund: www.frontierbcf.org
- Journal of Clinical Oncology: www.jcojournal.org
- National Action Plan on Breast Cancer: www.napbc.org
- National Alliance of Breast Cancer Organizations (NABCO): www.nabco.org
- The National Breast Cancer Coalition: www.natlbcc.org
- National Cancer Institute (NCI): www.nci.nih.gov
- ONCOLINK: www.oncolink.upenn.edu

Colon Health

Crohn's and Colitis Foundation of Canada
21 St. Clair Avenue East, Suite 301
Toronto, ON M4T 1L9
Tel: (416) 920-5035 or 1-800-387-1479
Fax: (416) 929-0364
e-mail: ccfc@cycor.ca

The Rudd Clinic for Diseases of the Colon and Rectum
123 Edward Street, Suite 825
Toronto, ON M5G 1E2
Tel: (416) 597-0997
Fax: (416) 597-2912
Web site:www.ruddclinic.com

Depression

Canadian Mental Health Association
2160 Yonge Street, 3rd Floor
Toronto, ON M4S 2Z3
Tel: (416) 484-7750
Fax: (416) 484-4617
e-mail: cmhanat@interlog.com

Canadian Psychiatric Association
237 Argyle Avenue, Suite 200
Ottawa, ON K2P 1B8
Tel: (613) 234-2815

Centre for Addiction and Mental Health
33 Russell Street
Toronto, ON M5S 2S1
Tel: (416) 595-6878
Fax: (416) 595-6881

Clarke Institute of Psychiatry
250 College Street
Toronto, ON M5T 1R8
Tel: (416) 979-2221
Web site: www.clarke-inst.on.ca

Mood Disorders

British Columbia

Mood Disorders Association of British Columbia
201–2730 Commercial Drive
Vancouver, BC V5N 5P4
Tel: 604-873-0103
Fax: 604-873-3095

Alberta

Depression and Manic Depression Association of Alberta
Box 6404
Edmonton, AB T5K 2J5
Tel: 1-888-757-7077
Fax: (403) 987-4596

Organization for Bipolar Affective Disorders Society
1019–7th Avenue SW
Calgary AB T2P 1A8
Tel: (403) 263-7408

Saskatchewan

Society for Depression and Manic-Depression in Saskatchewan Inc.
2526 Cumberland Avenue South
Saskatoon, SK STJ 2A2
Tel: (306) 343-7518

Manitoba

The Society for Depression and Manic Depression of Manitoba, Inc.
4–1000 Notre Dame Avenue
Winnipeg, MB R3E ON3
Tel: 1-800-263-1460 or (204) 786-0987
Fax: (204) 783-4898

Ontario

The Mood Disorders Association of Ontario and Toronto
40 Orchard View Blvd., Suite 222
Toronto, ON M4R 1B9
Tel: (416) 486-8046
Fax: (416) 486-8127

Mental Health Program Service
121 Kennedy Avenue, Suite 100
Toronto, ON M6R 3A9
Tel: (416) 763-2188
Fax: (416) 763-2199

Quebec
Association des dépressifs et des maniaco-dépressifs
801 rue Sherbrooke est, bureau 300
Montreal, QC H2L 1X7
Tel: (514) 529-7552
Helpline: (514) 529-5619
Fax: (514) 529-9877

Nova Scotia
Depressive and Manic Depressive Society of Nova Scotia
c/o 73 Howe Street
Sydney, NS B14 4T9
Tel: (902) 539-7179

Hotlines

Depression Information Resource & Education Centre (DIRECT)
1-888-557-5051, ext. 8000
Also visit DIRECT Web site: http://www-fhs.mcmaster.ca/direct

1-800-THERAPIST (1-800-843-7274)
(This is a referral resource.)

Diabetes

Canadian Diabetes Association
15 Toronto Street, Suite 800
Toronto, ON M5C 2E3
Tel: (416) 363-3373
Fax: (416) 363-3393

Provincial Offices
British Columbia/Yukon
1091 West 8th Ave.
Vancouver, BC V6H 2V3
Tel: (604) 732-1331 or 1-800-665-6526
Fax: (604) 732-8444

Manitoba
102-310 Broadway
Winnipeg, MB R3C 0S6
Tel: (204) 925-3800 or1-800-782-0175
Fax: (204) 949-0266

New Brunswick
165 Regent Street, Suite 3
Fredericton, NB E3B 7B4
Tel: (506) 452-9009 or 1-800-884-4232
Fax: (506) 455-4728

Newfoundland/Labrador
354 Water Street, Suite 217
St. John's, NF A1C 1C4
Tel: (709) 754-0953
Fax: (709) 754-0734

Nova Scotia
6080 Young Street, Suite 101
Halifax, NS B3K 5L2
Tel: (902) 453-4232
Fax: (902) 453-4440

Prince Edward Island
P.O. Box 133
Charlottetown, PEI C1A 7K2
Tel: (902) 894-3005
Fax: (902) 368-1928

Saskatchewan
104–2301 Avenue CN
Saskatoon, SK S7L 5Z5
Tel: (306) 933-4446 or 1-800-996-4446
Fax: (306) 244-2012

Association du Diabète du Quebec
Quebec Affiliate
5635 Sherbrooke Avenue East
Montreal, QC H1N 1A2
Tel: (514) 259-3422
Fax: (514) 259-9286

Alberta/NWT
Suite 1010, Royal Bank Building
10117 Jasper Ave. NW
Edmonton, AB T5J 1W8
Tel: (403) 423-1232 or 1-800-563-0032
Fax: (403) 423-3322

Food/Nutrition

The Canadian Dietetic Association
480 University Avenue, Suite 601
Toronto, ON M5G 1V2
Tel: (416) 596-0857
Fax: (416) 596-0603

Canadian Organic Growers Inc.
Box 6408, Station J
Ottawa, ON K2A 3Y6

National Institute of Nutrition
265 Carling Avenue
Ottawa, ON K1S 2E1
Tel: (613) 235-3355
Fax: (613) 235-7032
e-mail: nin@nin.ca

Heart Health

Heart and Stroke Foundation of Canada
222 Queen Street, Suite 1402
Ottawa, ON K1P 5V9
Tel: (613) 569-4361
Fax: (613) 569-3278
Web site: www.hsf.ca

Health Resource Centre
Tel: (416) 367-3313 or 1-800-267-6817
Fax: (416) 367-2844
e-mail: heart@web.net
Web site: www.web.net/heart/

Osteoporosis

Osteoporosis Society of Canada (OSC)
National Office
33 Laird Drive
Toronto, ON M4G 3S9
Tel: (416) 696-2663
Fax: (416) 696-2673
Tollfree: (English) 1-800-463-6842 or
(French) 1-800-977-1778
e-mail: osc@osteoporosis.ca
Web site: www.osteoporosis.ca

Note: to locate the self-help group closest to you, call your nearest chapter (see below) or 1-800-463-6842

Alberta
(403) 237-7022

British Columbia – OSTOP (an affilliate of OSC)
(604) 731-4997

Fredericton
(506) 455-3041

Manitoba
(204) 772-3498

Peel
(905) 615-7532

Peterborough
(705) 740-2776

Quebec
1-800-977-1778

Saskatchewan
(306) 931-2663

National Osteoporosis Foundation
1150 17th Street NW, Suite 500
Washington, DC 20036
Tel: 202-223-2226
Web site: www.nof.org

bibliography

Abraham, Caroline. "Tamoxifen trial halted early. Women can choose breast-cancer drug." *Globe and Mail*, April 7, 1998.

American Diabetes Association: "An Introduction to Oral Medications for Diabetes." Posted to: Diabetes.com, January 1999.

———. "Standards of Medical Care for Patients with Diabetes Mellitus." *Diabetes Care* 21, supplement 1, Clinical Practice Recommendations 1998.

———. "The United Kingdom Prospective Diabetes Study (UKPDS) for Type 2 Diabetes: What you need to know about the results of a long-term study." Posted to: www.diabetes.org/January 1999.

"Antibiotics in Animals: An Interview with Stephen Sundlof, D.V.M., Ph.D." Intl. Food Info. Council, 1100 Connecticut Ave. N.W., Ste. 430, Washington, D.C. 20036, 1997.

"Antidepressants' impact mainly from boost of getting treated, study suggests." Associated Press, July 20, 1998.

Antonucci T. et al. "Impaired glucose tolerance is normalized by treatment with the thiazolidinedione." *Diabetes Care*, vol. 20, issue 2: 188-93 (February 1997).

Apple, Rima D. (ed.). *Women, Health and Medicine in America: A Historical Handbook*. Rutgers Univ. Press, 1992.

Armstrong, David G., et al. San Antonio Treatment-based Classification System for Assessment and Care of Diabetic Feet. *J. of Am. Pod. Med. Assn*. 87, no. 7 (July 1996).

"Aspirin may protect your colon against cancer, too." *Ladies Home Journal*, March 1998:131.

Bailar, John C. III, and Heather Gornick. "Cancer Undefeated." *NEJMed*. 336(22):1569-74 (May 29, 1997).

Bartlett J.G. "Epidemiology and clinical aspects of antibiotic-associated colitis." Proceedings of the 2nd International Symposium on Anaerobes, June 22, 1985, Tokyo.

Bass, Brenda, Diane Pross, and Peter Bell. "Recruitment for breast screening in a rural practice: trial of a physician's letter of invitation." *Canadian Family Physician* 40:1730-39 (October 1994).

Batt, Sharon. *Patient No More: The Politics of Breast Cancer.* Charlottetown, PEI: gynergy books, 1994.

Beard, Mary K., and Lindsay R. Curtis. *Menopause and the Years Ahead*. Tuscon, Arizona: Fisher Books, 1988.

Behen, Madonna. "The new breast cancer test: the discovery of the breast cancer gene is a medical milestone...what you need to know." *Good Housekeeping*, April 1996.

Bellafante, Ginia, "Who put the 'me' in feminism?" *Time*, June 29, 1998.

Benedict S. et al. "Breast cancer detection by daughters of women with breast cancer." *Cancer Practice* 5:213–19 (July 1997).

Bequaert Holmes, Helen. "A Call to Heal Medicine" in *Feminist Perspectives in Medical Ethics*, edited by Helen Bequaert Holmes and Laura M. Purdy (Indiana University Press, 1992).

Berndl, Leslie. "Understanding Fat." *Diabetes Dialogue* 42, no.1 (Spring 1995).

Bernstein, Leslie, and Jennifer L. Kelsey. "Epidemiology and Prevention of Breast Cancer." Department of Health Research and Policy, Stanford Univ. and Dept. of Preventive Med., Univ. of Southern Calif. (1996): 47-67.

Bertell, Rosalie. "Links between ionizing radiation and breast cancer." Paper presented at the World Conference on Breast Cancer, July13-17, 1997, Kingston, Ontario.

"Black Women More Likely to Have More Aggressive Breast Tumors." Posted at: wysiwyg://26/http://www.mediconsult.com/women/news/ (December 20, 1998).

"Body Size a Breast Cancer Risk." *Am. J. of Epid.* 145(11):1011-19 (1997).

Bondy M., and C. Mastromarino. "Ethical issues of genetic testing and their implications in epidemiologic studies." *Annals of Epid.* 7: 363-66 (May 1997).

Bonen, Arent. "Fueling your tank." *Diabetes Dialogue* 42, no. 4 (Winter 1995).

Bove C.M. et al. "Presymptomatic and predisposition genetic testing: ethical and social considerations. *Semin Oncol Nurs* 13:135-40 (May 1997).

"Breakthrough Tamoxifen Study." Retrieved online from: http://www2.cancer.org/zine/001/001_05151998_0.html, January 5, 1999.

"Breast Cancer (Prognostics) Excess Gene Product May Serve As Marker." *Women's Health Weekly*, February 9, 1998.

"Breast Cancer and Abortion." *New Woman,* April 1997, p. 99.

"Breast Cancer Classification." Retrieved online from: http://breastdoctor.com/breast/cancer/class/htm (February 18, 1999).

"Breast Cancer." Retrieved online from: http://www.erinet.com/fnadoc/brest.htm January 25, 1999.

"Breast removal effective for women with high cancer risk, study finds." Posted to: http://cnn.com/HEALTH/9901/13/mastectomy.decision/ January 13, 1999.

Breen, Mary J. "Poverty and Ill Health." *The Healthsharing Book: Resources for Canadian Women*. Toronto: The Women's Press, 1985. p. 150.

Breggin, Peter R., and Ginger Ross Breggin. *Talking Back to Prozac*. New York: St. Martin's Press, 1994.

———. *Toxic Psychiatry*. New York: St. Martin's Press, 1991.

Brewster, Wendy. "New study challenges cancer, estrogen link." Reuters, March 29, 1997.

Brind, Joel *et al*. "Induced Abortion as an Independent Risk Factor for Breast Cancer." Dept. of Nat. Sci., City Univ. of New York, and Center for Biostatistics and Epidemiology and Dept. of Pharmacology, Penn. State Univ., 1996.

Brinton, Louise A. *et al*. "Body Size and Breast Cancer Risk Among Women Under Age 45 Years." *Am. J. of Epidem.* (1996): 698.

British Columbia Women's Community Consultation Report. "The Challenges Ahead for Women's Health." B.C. Women's Hospital and Health Centre Society, Vancouver, 1995.

Brody, J. *et al*. "Mapping the history of pesticide use in the Cape Cod Breast Cancer and Environment Study." Paper presented at the World Conference on Breast Cancer, July13-17, 1997, Kingston, Ontario.

Brody, Jane E. "Personal Health," *New York Times*, April 2, 1997.

———. "Scientist at work: Bruce N. Ames; Strong views on origins of cancer." *New York Times*, 5 July 1994, C1.

Burstow, Bonnie, and Don Weitz. *Shrink Resistant: The Struggle Against Psychiatry in Canada*. Vancouver: New Star Books, 1998.

———. "Women and Therapy." *The Healthsharing Book: Resources for Canadian Women*. Toronto: The Women's Press, 1985.

Bursztajn, Harold J., and Archie Brodsky. "Authenticity and autonomy in the managed-care era: forensic psychiatric perspectives." *J. of Clin. Ethics* 5, no. 3:237 (Fall, 1994).

Busby, Chris. "The current increase in breast cancer trend worldwide has its origin in ionizing radiation exposure to components of global weapons testing fallout." Paper presented at the World Conference on Breast Cancer, July13-17, 1997, Kingston, Ontario.

"Calcium supplements not equally effective." Reuters, December 27, 1999. *Am. J. of Therapeutics* 1999; 6:303-11, 313-21; and *J. of Clin. Pharma.* 1999;39:1-4.

"Calories Count In Colon Cancer Risk." *Am. J. of Epidem.* 1997; 145:199-210.

Canadian Hypertension Society. "High Blood Pressure and Drug Treatment." 1999.

Canadian Medical Association Journal and the Canadian Diabetes Association. 1998 clinical practice guidelines for the management of diabetes in Canada. Supplement to CMAJ 1998;159 (8 suppl).

"Cancer center studies link between dietary fat and breast cancer." *Cancer Researcher Weekly,* 28 February 1994: 8. Report on a Univ. of Calif., Irvine, study.

"A Cancer Gene Makes Colon Removal An Option." *New York Times*, March 19, 1997.

"Cancer In Massachusetts Town Caused By Demographics, Not Environment." *Boston Globe*, January 15, 1997.

Cancer Trials: Breast Cancer." Retrieved online from: http://207.121.187.155/NCI_CANCER_...ialInfo/Advances/breastCancer.html, January 25, 1999.

"Cancer-cell detection methods—breast cancer vaccine development." *Cancer Biotechnology Weekly,* 30 January 1995: 6.

Caplan L.S. "Disparities in breast cancer screening: is it ethical?" *Public Health Review* 25: 31-41 (1997).

Caplan, Paula J. *They Say You're Crazy: How the World's Most Powerful Psychiatrists Decide Who's Normal*. New York: Addison-Wesley Publishing Co., 1995.

"Carbohydrate Counting: A New Way to Plan Meals." American Diabetes Association. Posted to: Diabetes.com, January 1999.

Carroll, Rory. "Recovered Memory Techniques Are Bogus, Report Says." *The Guardian,* January 13, 1998.

Casciato, Dennis, and Barry B. Lowitz, eds. *Manual of Clinical Oncology, 2nd ed.*, (Boston: Little Brown, 1988).

Casper, Robert F., and Alcide Chapdelaine. "Estrogen and Interrupted Progestin: A New Concept for Menopausal Hormone Replacement Therapy," *Am. J. Obstet. and Gyn.* 168, April 1993.

Cass, Hyla. *St. John's Wort: Nature's Blues Buster.* New York: Avery Publishing Group, 1998.

Casstevens, Rebecca. "Addressing current uses of pesticides linked with breast cancer." Paper presented at the World Conference on Breast Cancer, July13-17, 1997, Kingston, Ontario.

Chaddock, Brenda. "Activity is key to diabetes health." *Cdn. Pharm. J.* March 1997.

———. "Foul Weather Fitness: The hardest part is getting started."*Cdn. Pharm. J.* March 1996.

———. "The Magic of Exercise." *Cdn. Pharm. J.* September 1995.

———. "The Right Way to Read a Label." *Cdn. Pharm. J.* May 1996.

———. "Blood-glucose testing: Keep up with the trend." *Cdn. Pharm. J.* September 1996:17.

Chang, Trina. "Simplifying Breast Cancer Diagnosis." *Am. Health,* April 1997, p. 18.

Chesler, Phyllis. *Women and Madness.* New York: Avon Books, 1972.

Chilvers, Clair. "Oral contraceptives and cancer." *Lancet* 344 (19 November 1994):1378.

"Cholesterol and Women." *HealthNews,* from the publishers of the *NEJM*, November 21, 1995.

Cicala, Roger S. *The Heart Disease Sourcebook.* Los Angeles: Lowell House, 1998.

Clarke, Bill. "Action Figures." *Diabetes Dialogue* 43, no. 3 (Fall 1996).

Clute, Eva. "Tamoxifen—Breast cancer preventive or human carcinogen: 1997 update." Paper presented at the World Conference on Breast Cancer, July13-17, 1997, Kingston, Ontario.

Colborn, Theo, John Peterson Myers, and Dianne Dumanoski. *Our Stolen Future.* New York: Dutton, 1996.

Colditz, Graham A., Kathleen M. Egan, and Meir J. Stampher. "Hormone Replacement Therapy and Risk of Breast Cancer: Results of Epidemiologic Studies." *Am. J. of Obstet. and Gyn.* 168, May 1993.

Coleman, Brenda C. "Breast cancer is rarer than previously thought." Associated Press, March 24, 1998.

"Combat job stress: Does work make you sick?" Retrieved online from: http://www.convoke.com/markjr/cjstress.html, February 12, 1999.

"A Complex Question of Odds: Hormones Versus No Treatment," *HealthFacts*, 18 (January 1993).

Coney, Sandra. *The Menopause Industry: How the Medical Establishment Exploits Women.* Hunter House, 1994.

Costin, Carolyn. *The Eating Disorder Sourcebook.* Los Angeles: Lowell House, 1996; and Chicago: Contemporary Books.

Cotton, Paul. "Environmental estrogenic agents area of concern." *JAMA* 271 (9 February 1994): 414, 416.

Cronier, Claire. "Sweetest Choices." *Diabetes Dialogue* 44, no. 1 (Spring 1997).

"Daughters of Breast Cancer Patients Need Help." *Medical Post,* 16 April 1996: 42.

Davis, D.L. *et al*. "Medical hypothesis: Xenoestrogens as preventable causes of breast cancer." *Environ. Health Prospect* 101, no. 5 (1993): 372–77.

Dawson, P. J. *et al*. "MCF10AT: A model for the evolution of breast cancer from proliferative breast disease." *Am. J. Pathol.*148, no. 1 January 1996): 313–19.

Dedyna, Katherine. "Cancer society exploring alternative therapy—Complementary medicine should have role in health care system, offical says," *Times Colonist*, May 6, 1997.

Delanet, Kathy, and Squillace, Marie. *Living with Heart Disease*. Los Angeles: Lowell House, 1998.

DeMarco, Carolyn. "Keys to the highway." *Wellness MD* 3, no. 6 (November/December 1993).

———. "Military research: Endometriosis and environmental toxins linked?" *Wellness MD* 4, no. 2 (March/April 1994): 23

———. "Preserving our environment: Breast cancer and the environment." *Health Naturally* 18 (October/November 1995): 26-30.

———. "The great mammogram debate: Are we spending millions to do naught for ought?" *Wellness MD* 3, no. 1 (January/February 1993).

———. *Take Charge of your Body: A Woman's Guide to Health*. Winlaw, B.C.: The Last Laugh, 1990.

Dickens, B.M. "The Doctrine of Informed Consent." In *Justice Beyond Orwell*, ed. Abella R. S. and M. L. Rothman. (Montreal: Yvon Blais, 1985) 243-63.

Dickens, Bernard M., Nancy Pei, and Kathryn M. Taylor. "Legal and Ethical Issues in Genetic Testing and Counselling for Susceptibility to Breast, Ovarian and Colon Cancer." *Cdn Med. Assoc. J.* March 15, 1996; 154 (6):813-18.

"Diet and breast cancer." *Nutrition Research Newsletter,* vol. 13 (September 1994): 101. Adapted from *Archives Internal Medicine,* August 22, 1994, and *British J. Cancer*, September 1994.

Doan, Brian D. et al. "Psychological issues facing high risk women seeking genetic testing for hereditary breast cancer." Paper presented at the World Conference on Breast Cancer, July13-17, 1997, Kingston, Ontario.

Doepel, Laurie, K. "Looking at Menopause's Role in Osteoporosis," *JAMA* 254, no. 17, November 1, 1985.

Dolinger, Ernest H., M. D. Rosenbaum, and Greg Cable. *Everyone's Guide To Cancer Therapy*. Toronto: Somerville House, 1995.

Doress, Paula Brown, Diana Laskin Siegal, and the Midlife and Older Women Book Project in Cooperation with the Boston Women's Health Collective. *Ourselves Growing Older*. New York: Simon and Schuster 1987.

"Double mastectomy cuts breast cancer risk by 90 percent: study." Posted online to: http://www/yahoo/com/sg/headlines/...6316820-90114132720.newsworld.html, January 14, 1999.

Dreher, Henry, and Alice D. Domar. *Healing Mind, Healthy Woman.* New York: Henry Holt and Co. 1996.

Drum, David, and Terry Zierenberg. *The Type 2 Diabetes Sourcebook.* Los Angeles: Lowell House 1998.

Dunn, Bruce. "The Israeli Breast Cancer Anomaly." *abreast* 1, no. 4 (Winter 95-96):5.

"Exercise and Breast Cancer—Time to Get Moving? *NEJM*, 336, no.18 (May 1, 1997).

Elmore Joann G. *et al.* "Variability in radiologists' interpretations of mammograms." *NEJM* 331, no. 22 (1 December 1994): 1493-99.

Emanuel, Ezekiel J., and Linda L. Emanuel. "Four models of the physician-patient relationship." *JAMA* 1992, 267 (16): 2221-26.

Engel, June V. "Beyond Vitamins: Phytochemicals to help fight disease." *Health News* 14. (June 1996) Univ. of Toronto.

Engel, June. *The Complete Breast Book.* Toronto: Key Porter Books, 1996.

———. "Eating Fibre." *Diabetes Dialogue,* vol. 44, no. 1 (Spring 1997).

"Engineering a treatment for Crohn's disease." *Lancet*, vol. 349, no. 9051, 22 February 1997.

"EPA to study safety of an insecticide." *New York Times,* 24 October 1993:10.

Epstein, Samuel S. "Pesticides pose a lifelong threat." *New York Times,* 29 August 1994, p.14.

Epstein, Samuel S., David Steinmean, with Suzanne LeVert. *The Breast Cancer Prevention Program: The First Complete Survey of the Causes of Breast Cancer and the Steps You Can Take to Reduce Your Risks.* New York: Macmillan, 1998.

Esserman, Dr. Laura. "Breast cancer gene screening for at-risk women." Posted online at: http://mediconsult.com/breast/news/, November 8, 1998.

"Estimating Breast Cancer Risk." National Cancer Institute bulletins. Posted online to: http://cancernet.nci.nih.gov/clinp...Estimating_Breast_Cancer_Risk.html, December 1998.

"Estrogen Gene Tied To Breast Cancer Risk." *New York Times*, March 26, 1997.

"Estrogen Replacement Therapy and Breast Cancer Risk." *Cancer Researcher Weekly*, May 10, 1993.

Etchells, E. *et al.* "Disclosure." *CMAJ* 1996, 155:387-91.

———. "Voluntariness." *CMAJ* 1996, 155:1083-86.

———. "Consent." *CMAJ* 1996, 155:177-80.

"Evaluation of a breast mass." *NEJM* 328:810-12 (1993).

Evans, Richard A. "Breast conserving surgery: Is radiation therapy always necessary?" Paper presented at the World Conference on Breast Cancer, July13-17, 1997, Kingston, Ontario.

"Everyday Carcinogens: Stopping Cancer Before It Starts." Proceedings from the March 1999 workshop on primary cancer prevention, McMaster Univ., Hamilton, Ontario.

"Evidence for Estrogen." *Medical Post,* 9 April 1996: 75-76.

Evista patient information. Eli Lilly and Co., Indianapolis, 1999.

"FDA approves first blood test for breast cancer recurrence." Retrieved online from http://208.206.43.181/womens/T96-22.html, January 5, 1999.

Feig, S.A. "Estimation of currently attainable benefit from mammographic screening of women aged 40-49 years." *Cancer* 75: 2412-19, no. 1186 (1995).

Feldman, Gayle. "Is Genetic Testing Right For You?" *Self.* October 1996:187-209.

Ferraro, Cathleen. "New Uses of Chemicals Linked To More Illness." Published online, Scripps-McClatchy Western, December 10, 1997.

Ferraro, Susan. "The anguished politics of breast cancer." *New York Times Mag.* 15 August 1993: 24.

Findlay, Deborah, and Leslie Miller. "Medical power and women's bodies." In B.S. Bolaria and R. Bolaria, eds. *Women, Medicine and Health* (1994, Fernwood, Halifax).

Finley, Don. "New breast cancer drug described as promising," *Winnipeg Free Press,* September 20, 1997.

Finucane, Fanchon F. "Decreased Risk of Stroke among Postmenopausal Hormone Users: Results From A National Cohort," *JAMA* vol. 269, June 2, 1993.

Fletcher, Suzanne W. "Confusion about Breast-Cancer Screening." *NEJM* 1997; 336:1465-71.

"Following the Patient With Chronic Disease." *Patient Care Canada,* vol. 7, no. 5, May 1996: 22-38.

"Food alone can't always provide requisite nutrition." *Globe and Mail,* September 28, 1998.

Food and Drug Administration. "Nutrient Claims Guide for Individual Foods." Special Report, Focus On Food Labeling. FDA Publication no. 95-2289.

Fugh-Berman, Adriane. *Alternative Medicine: What Works.* Tucson: Odonian Press, 1996.

"Garlic acts as an anti-carcinogen in breast cancer." *Cancer Researcher Weekly,* Report on two Penn. Sate Univ. studies 17 January 1994: 3.

Gilbert, Susan. "Doctors often misread results of genetic tests, study finds," *New York Times,* March 26, 1997.

Gills, A.M. "Research update: From the Washington, D.C., meeting on estrogens in the environment: global health implications." *Bioscience,* vol. 44, no. 5: 296–98.

Gordon, Dennis. "Acarbose: When it Works/ When it Doesn't." *Diabetes Forecast,* February 1997.

Greenberg, Brigitte, "Stress Hormone Linked To High-Fat Snacking In Women." Associated Press. April 4, 1998.

Greenpeace. *Body of Evidence: The Effects of Chlorine on Human Health*. 1994.

Greenwood, Sadja. *Menopause Naturally: Preparing for the Second Half of Life.* California: Volcano Press, 1992.

Habib, Marlene. "Low-fat diet and exercise reduce breast cancer risk." The Canadian Press, January 10, 1997.

———. "Pollution seen as chief culprit in breast cancer: 80 per cent of cases tied to ecology mishaps." *Winnipeg Free Press*, July 17, 1997.

Harvey, Robin. "Bras and breast cancer." *Toronto Star*, 18 March 1996.

"Health Monitor: Breast Cancer—Trans fatty acids may trigger the disease." *USA Today,* February 1998.

Henderson, I. Craig. "Paradigmatic shifts in the management of breast cancer." *NEJM* vol. 332, no. 14 (6 April 6 1995): 951-52.

Hendler, Saul Sheldon. *The Doctors' Vitamin and Mineral Encyclopedia,* New York: Fireside Books, 1990.

Hendren, John. "Popular herbal remedy reportedly fails potency tests." Associated Press, August 31, 1998.

Henkel, Gretchen. *Making the Estrogen Decision*. Los Angeles: Lowell House, 1992.

"High levels of saturated fat found to promote ovarian cancer." *New York Times*, 21 September 1994.

Highfield, Roger. "Gender-bending chemicals may cause cancers." *Daily Telegraph,* London, 26 July 1995, p.4.

Hilts, Philip. "Risks of Colon Cancer." *New York Times*, April 24, 1997.

Hislop, Gregory T. "The Role of Nutrition in the Prevention of Cancer." *Cdn J. of CME* March 1995:111-18.

Ho, Marian. "Learning Your ABCs, Part Two." *Diabetes Dialogue,* vol. 43, No. 3 (Fall 1996).

Holowaty, Phillippa. "Breast Cancer Gene Research." Presented to Alliance of Breast Cancer Survivors, November 13, 1997.

Holtzman N.A. "Medical and ethical issues in genetic screening—an academic view." *Environ. Health Perspect.* 1996 Oct 104 Suppl 5: 987-90.

Horsman, Doug. "Hereditary Cancer Testing and Counselling in BC." *abreast*, vol. 1, no. 4 (Winter 95-96):4-8.

"How to deal with stress." Retrieved online from: http://www.backrelief.com/stress.htm, February 12, 1999.

Howe, Geoffrey, R. "Dietary Fat and Breast Cancer Risks." *Cancer Supplement*, vol. 74, no. 3, August 1, 1994.

Hoy, Claire, *The Truth About Breast Cancer*. Toronto: Stoddart Publishing, 1995.

Hufnagel, Vicki. *No More Hysterectomies*. New York: New American Library, 1989.

"IFIC Review: Intense Sweeteners: Effects on Appetite and Weight Management." Intl. Food Info. Council, 1100 Connecticut Ave. N.W., Ste. 430, Washington, D.C. 20036, November 1995.

"IFIC Review: Uses and Nutritional Impact of Fat Reduction Ingredients." Intl. Food Info. Council, 1100 Connecticut Ave. N.W., Ste. 430, Washington, D.C. 20036, October 1995.

Immen, Wallace. "Five promising finds in the fight against cancer." *Globe and Mail*, April 30, 1997.

———. "Repeated dieting may raise cancer risk. Chemicals stored in fat spur rapid growth and may increase chances of mutations in cells." *Globe and Mail*, April 16, 1997.

Jamison, Kay Redfield. *An Unquiet Mind: A Memoir of Moods and Madness*. New York: Vintage Books, 1995.

Joffe, Russell, M.D., and Anthony Levitt. *Conquering Depression*. Hamilton: Empowering Press, 1998.

Johnson, Catherine. *When to Say Goodbye to Your Therapist*. New York: Simon and Schuster, 1988.

Kolata, Gina. "Ticking Bomb The Presence of a Breast-Cancer Gene Creates Other Problems For Some Women." *New York Times*, Sunday, March 2, 1997.

———. "Another Group Switches on Frequency of Mammograms." *New York Times*, March 28, 1997.

Kopans, Daniel B. "The accuracy of mammographic interpretation." *NEJM,* vol. 331, no. 22 (1 December 1994): 1521-22.

Kra, J. Siegfried. *What Every Woman Must Know About Heart Disease*. New York: Warner Books, 1996.

Lawless, O.J. *et al*. "Silicone-specific T-cell reactivity in saline breast implants and non-breast implant patients." Retrieved online from: http://www.geocity.com/Hotsprings/8689/saline/s08.html, January 19, 1999.

LeBlanc, Gerald A. *"Are Environmental Sentinels Signaling?" Environ. Health Perspec.*, vol. 103, no. 10, October 1995.

Lee, John R. *What Your Doctor May Not Tell You About Menopause*. New York: Warner Books, 1996.

Leibenluft, Ellen. "Why are so may women depressed?" *Women's Health* vol. 9, no.2 (Summer, 1998).

Leiter, Lawrence A. "Acarbose:New Treatment In NIDDM Patients." *New Drugs/Drug News*, vol. 14, no. 2. Ontario College of Pharmacists.

Lemonick, Michael D. "Eat your heart out." *Time*, 19 July 1999.

Lembo, Anthony, ed. IBS and Crohn's-Colitis FAQ. Posted to the Internet as alt.support.crohns-colitis and alt.support.ibs. E-mail queries to alembo@UCLA.edu or juniper@uiuc.edu, 1996.

Leutwyler, Kristin. "Dying to be thin." *Women's Health,* vol. 9, no. 2 (Summer, 1998).

Linton, Marilyn. *Taking Charge by Taking Care*. Toronto: Macmillan Canada, 1996.

Long, Patricia. "More than 90 percent of women diagnosed with early breast cancer survive." *Health Magazine*, 1995, Document mpl395c.

Love, Susan. *Dr. Susan Love's Breast Book, 2nd Ed.* New York City: Addison-Wesley, 1995.

Lubin, F. "A case-control study of caffeine and methylxanthines in benign breast disease." *JAMA*, 1985, no. 196; 253:2388-92.

MacRae, Paul. "Margaret Wente—Opinion—Finally: a piece of good news in the breast cancer debate." *Times Colonist*, March 25, 1997.

"Major causes of ill health." *Rachel's Environment & Health Weekly #584*. Published online by the Environmental Research Foundation. February 2, 1998.

"Mammogram Screening by Specialists vs. 'General' Radiologists." Posted online at: wysiwyg://26/http://www.mediconsult.com/women/news/, December 22, 1998.

Mangano, Joseph J. "Breast cancer from radioactive emissions by nuclear power plants in Connecticut, USA." Paper presented at the World Conference on Breast Cancer, July13-17, 1997, Kingston, Ontario.

Mattila, Antti. "Life At The Crossroads: Depression—Philosophical Perspectives." Paper presented at The Fourth International Conference on Philosophical Practice, August 3-7, 1998, Bergisch Gladbach, Germany.

McAuliffe, Kathleen. "Dying Of Embarrassment." *More*, May/June, 1999:52-62.

McKay, John. "Breast Health—Seaweed cited as factor in low cancer rates in Japan." *Times Colonist*, September 9, 1997.

National Institutes of Health Consensus Statement. Breast cancer screening for women ages 40-49, January 21-23, 1997. Bethesda: National Cancer Institute, 1997.

"New Evidence: Drug Halves Breast-Cancer Rate. Study Shows Tamoxifen May Prevent Breast Cancer." Posted online to: http://www.newsnet5.com/yourhealth/yourhealth-980915-182736.html, September 15, 1998.

"New study challenges cancer, estrogen link." *Times Colonist,* March 29, 1997.

Newcomb, P.A. *et al*. "Pregnancy termination in relation to risk of breast cancer." *JAMA,* vol. 275, no. 4 (24-31 January 1996): 283-87.

———. "Lactation and a reduced risk of premenopausal breast cancer." *NEJM,* vol. 330, no. 2 (13 January 1994): 81-87.

"Numerous roadblocks keeping botanicals across border." *Globe and Mail,* September 28, 1998.

"Nutrients in fruit and vegetables linked to bone health, Reuters, Jan. 4, 2000. (Source: *Am. Jour. of Clin. Nutrition* 2000;71:142-51).

O'Connell, Peter, et al. "Molecular genetic studies of early breast cancer evolution by LOH." Retrieved online from: http://mars.uthscsa.edu/Publications/MGSEBCE/mgse-bce.html, February 16, 1999.

"Olestra: yes or no?" Excerpted from the Univ. of California at Berekley Wellness Letter, c. Health Associates, 1996 in *Diabetes Dialogue,* vol. 43, no. 3 (Fall 1996).

"OncoLink Cancer News: Breast cancer risk reduced after bilateral prophylactic mastectomy in high-risk patients," Reuters, January 14, 1999.

"OncorMed Granted Patent For BRCA1 Gene Sequence." *Cancer Economics*, vol. 12 no. 8, (August 1997).

Ontario Task Force on the Primary Prevention of Cancer. Recommendations for the Primary Prevention of Cancer: Report of the Ontario Task Force on the Primary Prevention of Cancer.[Toronto]: March 1995. Presented to the Ontario Ministry of Health.

"Osteoporosis Drug Has Added Benefit of Lowering Breast Cancer Risk." Posted online to: http://mediconsult.com/breast/news/, December 18, 1998.

Osteoporosis Society of Canada. "Biophosphates." Fact Sheet Series Number 9, 1999.

———. "Cacitonin: Its Role in the Treatment of Osteoporosis." Press Release, November 1999.

———. "Calcium." Fact Sheet Series Number 3, 1999.

———. "Hormone Therapy." Fact Sheet Series Number 8, 1999.

———. "How Strong Are Your Bones." Fact Sheet Series Number 4, 1999.

———. "Living With Osteoporosis." Fact Sheet Series Number 1, 1999

———. "SERMS: Their role in the Prevention of Osteoporosis." Press Release, December 1998.

Patlak, Margie. "Estrogens May Link Pesticides, Breast Cancer." *Environ. Sci. and Tech. / News* 5 (vol. 143, 1996): 210, 211.

Perry, Susan, and Katherine O'Hanlan. *Natural Menopause: The Complete Guide to a Woman's Most Misunderstood Passage*. New York: Addison-Wesley Publishing, Inc., 1992.

Plotkin, David. "Good News and Bad News about Breast Cancer." *Atlantic Monthly,* June 1996, 53-82.

Poirier, Laurinda, and Katharine M. Coburn. *Women & Diabetes: Life Planning for Health and Wellness.* New York: Amer. Diabetes Assoc. and Bantam Books, 1997.

"Preventive mastectomy: an option for high-risk women." Posted online to: http://sss.mayohealth.org/mayo/9901/htm/breastop.htm, January 13, 1999.

"Prozac: help or hype?" *Health for Women,* vol. VIII, no. 2 (Spring/Summer, 1998).

Quinn, Brian P. *The Depression Sourcebook.* Los Angeles: Lowell House and Contemporary Books, Chicago, 1997.

Raloff, J.A. "Plastics may shed chemical estrogens." *Science News,* vol. 144 (3 July 1993): 12.

———. "Ecocancers." *Science News,* vol. 144 (3 July 1993): 10-13.

———. "Menstrual cycles may affect cancer risk." *Science News,* vol. 147 (7 January 1995): 7.

———. "Obesity, diet linked to breast cancer." *Science News,* vol. 147 (21 January 1995): 39.

Ramlow, J.M., G.W. Olsen, and G.G. Bond. "Environment health link calls for study." *Environ. Prot.* vol. 5, no. 9 (1994): 63-68.

Rampe, David. "Losing Pounds by Surfing on the Web." *New York Times*, December 7, 1999, 8.

Randolph, Laura B. "Confronting a Major Killer of Black Women: A Save-your-life Guide." *Ebony,* October 1997.

Rebbeck T.R., *et al*. "Genetic heterogeneity in hereditary breast cancer: role of BRCA1 and BRCA2." *Am J Hum Genet*. 1996 59(3): 547-53.

Recer, Paul. "Women Hurt More, In More Places, But Cope Better, Studies Say." Associated Press, April 7, 1998.

Reilly P.R. *et al*. "Ethical issues in genetic research: disclosure and informed consent." *Nat Genet* 1997 Jan 15:16-20.

"Return of Crohn's." *The Lancet*, vol. 349, no. 9053, 8 March 1997.

Rifkin, Jeremy. "Playing God with the Genetic Code." *Health Naturally,* April/May 1995: 40-44.

Roberts, Felicia D. *et al*. "Self-reported stress and risk of breast cancer." Retrieved online at: Does Stress Really Cause Breast Cancer? Stop Worrying Says New Study. Posted online to: www.mediconsul...urnal/automation/960102061018.html , February 18, 1999.

Robson, Barbara. "Conferences Point to Growing Concern about Possible Links Between Breast Cancer, Environment." *Can. Med. Assoc. J.* 8 (154; 15 April 1996): 1254.

Rosenberg, L. *et al*. "Case-control study of oral contraceptive use and risk of breast cancer." *Am. J. Epidem.,* vol. 143, no. 1 (1 January 1996): 25-37.

Roth, Loren H., Meisel, Alan, and Lidz, Charles W. "Tests of Competency to Consent to Treatment." *Amer. Jour. Psych.* (vol. 134, no. 4) 1977.

Rowley, Peter T. "Confusion about Breast Cancer Screening." *NEJM* 1997; 336:1465-71.

Rudd, Wm. Warren. *Advice From The Rudd Clinic: A Guide To Colorectal Health.* Toronto: Macmillan Canada, 1997.

Safe, Stephen H. "Xenoestrogens and Breast Cancer" *NEJM*, vol. 337, no. 18 (October 30, 1977).

Schrag D. *et al*. " Decision analysis—effects of prophylactic mastectomy and oophorectomy on life expectancy among women with BRCA1 or BRCA2 mutations." *NEJM*, 1997 336 (20):1465.

Schreiber, Tatiana. "Misleading and Irresponsible: Cancer Activists Decry Harvard Report," *Resist,* April 1997.

"Scientific study explores role of dietary fat in breast cancer." Retrieved online from: http://www.media.wayne.edu/iws.back.issues/iws3_20_97/breast_cancer.html, January 5, 1999.

Seto, Carol. "Nutrition Labelling—U.S. style." *Diabetes Dialogue,* The Canadian Diabetes Association (Vol. 42, No.1) Spring 1995.

Sierpina, Diane. "Making Strides Against Breast Cancer." *New York Times*, October 25, 1998.

"Sorting Out the Facts About Fat." Intl. Food Info. Council, 1100 Connecticut Ave. N.W., Ste. 430, Washington, D.C. 20036,1997.

Soto, Ana M., Kerrie L. Chung, and Carlos Sonnenschein. "The Pesticides Endosulfan, Toxaphene, and Dieldrin Have Estrogenic Effets on Human Estrogen-Sensitive Cells." *Environ. Health Perspec.*, vol 102, February 1994.

Spake, Amanda. "Our Worst Fears About Pesticides And Plastics May Be Coming True—If Maverick Researcher Devra Lee Davis Is Right." 1995 *HEALTH magazine*, Document ID: MASO95C.

Sponselli, Christina. "Genetic testing raises questions." *Nurseweek*, November 1997.

———. "RNs can answer questions about genetics." *Nurseweek*, November 1997.

Steinberg, W.M. "Menopause and breast cancer." *Patient Care,* May 1993: 8. Letter.

Steingraber, Sandra. *Living Downstream: An Ecologist Looks At Cancer and the Environment*. New York: Addison-Wesley, 1997.

"Stress." Retrieved online from: http://meagherlab.tamu.edu/M-Meagher/Abnormal/stressout.htlm, February 12, 1999.

"Study Further Links Smoking To Depression." Reuters, February 10, 1998.

"Study: Breast Self-Exam May Not Save Lives." Reuters, Tuesday March 4, 1997.

Thornton, Joe. "Chlorine, human health and the environment: The breast cancer warning." Washington, D.C.: Greenpeace, 1993. A report prepared for Greenpeace.

Thune, Inger *et al*. "Physical Activity and the Risk of Breast Cancer." *NEJM*, vol. 336, no. 18:1269-75 (May 1, 1997).

"To Test Or Not To Test: The Debate Over Cancer-Gene Testing." *Salt Lake Tribune*, Feb 11, 1997.

"Update on the Ontario Task Force on the Primary Prevention of Cancer." City of Toronto Public Health Department, May 16, 1996.

Weber, Barbara L. "Clinical implications of basic research: Susceptibility genes for breast cancer." *NEJM,* vol. 331, no. 22 (1 December 1994): 1523-24.

Webster, Katharine. "Remove breasts, lengthen life? Studies examine gene mutations." Canadian Press, May 15, 1997.

Weed, Susun S., *Wise Woman Ways: Menopausal Years.* New York: Ash Tree Publishing, 1992.

———. *Menopausal Years: The Wise Woman Way—Alternative Approaches for Women* 30-90. New York: Ash Tree Publishing, 1992.

Whiteford, Linda. "Political economy, gender and the social production of health and illness." In C. Sargent and C. Brettell, eds. *Gender and Health.* Toronto: Prentice-Hall, 1996.

Willett, W.C. et al. "Intake of Trans Fatty Acids and Risk of Coronary Heart Disease Among Women." *Lancet* 341:581-5, 1993.

———. "Prospective studies of Diet and Breast Cancer." *Cancer Supplement*, vol. 74, no. 3, August 1, 1994.

Williams, Linda S., "International Conference on Reproductive and Genetic Engineering and Women's Reproductive Health." *Resources for Feminist Research*, vol. 18, no. 3, 1989.

"Women Find Themselves Courted By Pharmaceutical Firms." Associated Press, July 20, 1998.

Wright, Jonathan V., and John Morgenthaler. *Natural Hormone Replacement.* (Petaluma, CA: Smart Publications, 1997.

"Younger Women React Differently Than Older Women to Mastectomies." Posted online to: http://mediconsult.com/breast/news/, December 4, 1998.

"Your medical test guide." *Health for Women,* vol. VIII, no. 2 (Spring/Summer, 1998).

Index